MW01041851

Respiratory Home Care Equipment

Steven P. McPherson, R.R.T.

Raul Ospina

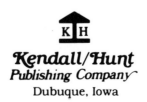

Kendall/Hunt Publishing Company

Dubuque, Iowa

Dedication

This book is dedicated to my
great support staff: Punk,
Monkey, and Squirrel.

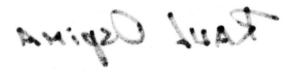

Library of Congress Catalog Card Number: 87–82074

ISBN 0–8403–4527–5

Printed in the United States of America
10 9 8 7 6 5 4 3 2 1

Contents

Preface

The fastest growing subspecialty in Respiratory Care is the area of Home Care. With the onset of prospective payment systems, hospitals are discharging patients sooner. And as critical care measures have improved patient survival, patients are being discharged with a larger variety and complexity of disorders. Many of these patients do not have stabilized disease processes and are much more difficult to manage than the patient in the home of days gone by. Certainly these patients can be a significant challenge to the Respiratory Home Care Provider. Because of more complicated home care patient problems, the Respiratory Care Practitioner must be well versed in the therapy and apparatus required to individualize and maximize the patient's care.

Quality home care for these patients not only allows the patient to be in the familiar surroundings of his/her home, but substantially reduces the financial burden on the family as compared to long term hospitalization. With the patient's regime individualized and closely monitored, the quality of life can be dramatically improved with the patient in his/her own surroundings and repeat hospital admissions can be minimized. This also requires the Practitioner to be familiar with cleaning, disinfection, and surveillance procedures to minimize recurrent bouts of infection.

The Respiratory Care Practitioner is also, of course, the patient and family educator. It is the practitioner's role to make certain that all individuals involved in the patient's care be thoroughly familiar with the equipment, therapy, assessment of the patient, and all safety precautions. All family members must have enough basic knowledge to be alert for problems with the patient and the equipment in use.

The single most dramatic change in Respiratory Home Care is the increase in patients being discharged to their home on ventilators. The home care ventilator patient now also covers all age groups, requiring the Respiratory Therapist to have a thorough background in the variety of disease processes and ventilator management techniques along with a thorough knowledge of the variety of ventilators and associated equipment required to provide ventilatory life support in the home.

As described above, the challenge facing the Respiratory Home Care Practitioner is a complicated one and I hope that the contents of the text will help you face that challenge.

Steven P. McPherson

Acknowledgment

The author wishes to deliver a special thanks to Ray Masferrer and Sherry Milligan for all their hard work and help on this project. In addition, I would like to thank Sam Giordano for his support and encouragement, along with all the manufacturers for their help.

1 *Gas Delivery Devices*

Nearly all respiratory home care devices require a source of gas. The gas may be the primary form of therapy, such as with the administration of oxygen, or the gas may be required to power another device. The respiratory care practitioner must have a thorough knowledge of gas delivery systems in order to best meet the patient's individual needs. The patient and family should be familiarized with the patient's system, as well, so they can feel comfortable with its operation and can respond correctly in the event of problems.

Cylinders

Liquid Carbonics of General Dynamics introduced the first medical gas cylinders in 1888.[1] Prior to that time, oxygen was produced at the site of its administration, either through chemical methods or by electrolysis of water. This made oxygen therapy cumbersome and long-term therapy impossible. Cylinders greatly enhanced the availability of oxygen and other gases, such as compressed air. A variety of small cylinders are now available from Mada, Ventco, Erie, UOE, S.L.O., Puritan-Bennett and Western Enterprises, which provides the Home Care Practitioner with a variety of options for each patient.

Regulation of Construction and Transport

Regulation of cylinder construction was moved from the Interstate Commerce Commission (ICC) to the Department of Transportation (DOT) in 1967, and all cylinders were required to meet DOT standards by the beginning of 1970.[2] The regulatory jurisdiction is divided between subdivisions of the Department of Transportation: The Federal Highway Administration regulates road transport of cylinders, the Federal Railroad Administration is responsible for rail transport, the Federal Aviation Administration (FAA) governs air transport, and the United States Coast Guard regulates the transport of cylinders in U.S. waters.[2]

A patient requiring oxygen during travel should contact his physician for considerations about or changes to be made in oxygen delivery. Arrangements should be made well in advance with the airline, rail, bus, or shipline company. Most companies can make provisions for patients requiring oxygen, but airlines are required by the FAA to use only oxygen equipment that they maintain, underscoring the need for arrangements to be made in advance. Bus and rail companies will allow patients to use their own oxygen equipment, but again advance arrangements must be made. Most companies require a physician order; some will require a release letter and may wish to contact the patient's physician. The patient should be instructed to request seating in a no-smoking area. If planning to travel by car, the patient must know how to estimate his oxygen usage, should plan the trip around oxygen refill points, and should be mindful of the need for adequate ventilation in the car to prevent an accumulation of excessive oxygen concentrations. The safety precautions described in this chapter regarding ignition sources, combustible materials, and mechanical hazards apply during travel as well as at home.

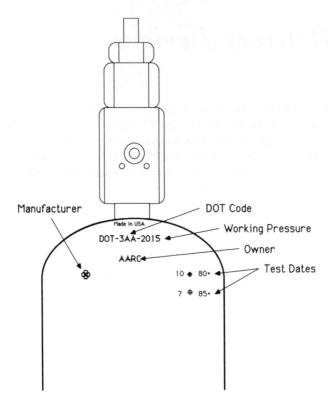

Figure 1.1 Cylinder markings.

Cylinder Markings and Labeling

There are a number of cylinder markings that provide information (Figure 1.1). The DOT (or ICC) marking on the cylinder indicates that standards were met at the time the cylinder was constructed.[2] The code following the DOT marking indicates the type of material used in the cylinder's construction. The notation "3A" indicates that the cylinder is of a high-carbon steel or medium-manganese steel, "3AA" means that the steel was heat-treated, and "3AL" signifies an aluminum cylinder.[3] The next set of numbers following the DOT code is the approved working pressure for that cylinder. The DOT allows cylinders to be filled 10% higher than the working pressure to take into account pressure variations due to ambient temperature changes. The manufacturer's mark and the country where the cylinder was manufactured are stamped onto the cylinder along with the original hydrostatic test date. DOT requires that most cylinders be hydrostatically tested initially and every 5 years thereafter to assess the expansion characteristics and, therefore, the safety of the cylinder. Some high-strength steel cylinders are required to be retested only every 10 years, a fact that is indicated by a star following the DOT-3 code. At retesting, both an internal and an external visual inspection is completed, and a plus sign following the retest date indicates that the cylinder passed both inspections. (Aluminum cylinders *do not* have a plus sign following the retest date.) The test facility's mark is also included with the retest date. An ownership mark and serial number may also be present. All cylinders must contain a pressure release mechanism approved by the Bureau of Explosives.[2] The release is usually a diaphragm that does not reseat and is designed to rupture in the presence of excessive pressure or temperature.

The labeling required for medical gas cylinders was designed by the Compressed Gas Association (CGA) and adopted by the American Standards Association. The international symbol for the gas contents (**"AIR"** for compressed air and **"O₂"** for oxygen) must be displayed along with the name of the gas in the language of the country in which the cylinder was filled. The federal Food and Drug Administration (FDA) requires that the gas meet minimum purity standards (99.0% for oxygen) and that the purity figure must be stated on the label as listed in the United States Pharmacopeia (USP) or National Formulary (NF).[4] The label must be easily visible and must not conflict with DOT labeling or color codes. An alert to the potential hazards, including the fact that the contents are under high pressure, should be displayed, along with instructions on how to deal with the hazards. The supplier must keep records of the lot numbers of the gases supplied to each patient.

Color-Coding System

A color-coding system was also designed by the CGA and later adopted by the Bureau of Standards. The color code for oxygen in the United States is *green,* although patients traveling outside the U.S. should be informed that the international color code for oxygen is *white.* Air is usually color coded yellow or black and green (black being the designated color for nitrogen and green for oxygen, the primary components of air). Helium's designated color code is brown, so helium/oxygen mixtures are color coded brown and green. Color codes provide a visual indicator only, and the label should be checked before any cylinder gas is administered to a patient. If the label is not intact or if there is a conflict between the color code and label, the cylinder should not be used.

Valve Indexing

The cylinder valve acts as a needle valve in opening and closing the cylinder (Figure 1.2). The valve also contains the pressure release mechanism previously described. Large cylinder handwheel-type valves are indexed according to a system developed by the CGA and refined and approved by the American Standards Association.[4] The American Standard indexing uses the threads and nipple of the connection (Figure 1.3) to index each gas connection differently for life-support and non-life-sustaining equipment. Left-handed and internal threaded connections are reserved for non-life-supporting gases. Adapters that allow a change from one gas connection to another should not be used.

Small cylinder post-type valves are indexed by a system that employs two pins and correspondingly located holes, called the Pin Index Safety System. Figure 1.4 shows the design of the pin index system. Devices that have had the pins removed should not be used until the pins are properly replaced.

Indexing of Outlet Connections

The CGA also designed an indexing system for the outlet connections of devices that are connected to cylinders. The Diameter Index Safety System (DISS) uses the threads and the nipple configuration to index the outlets of lower pressure devices, a system similar to the American

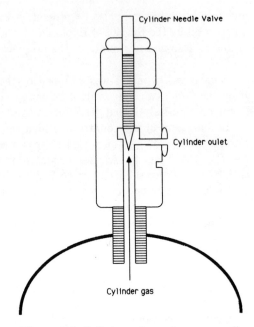

Figure 1.2 Cylinder valve acts as a needle valve to open and close the cylinder.

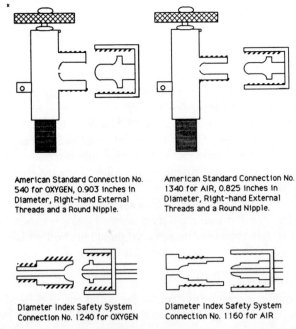

American Standard Connection No. 540 for OXYGEN, 0.903 Inches In Diameter, Right-hand External Threads and a Round Nipple.

American Standard Connection No. 1340 for AIR, 0.825 Inches In Diameter, Right-hand External Threads and a Round Nipple.

Diameter Index Safety System Connection No. 1240 for OXYGEN

Diameter Index Safety System Connection No. 1160 for AIR

Figure 1.3 American Standard and Diameter Index Safety System Connections.

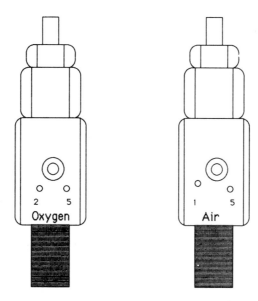

Figure 1.4 Pin Index Safety System for oxygen and air used on small cylinders with post type valves.

Standard indexing for high pressure cylinder valve outlets. Figure 1.4 shows the DISS indexing for air and oxygen.

Safety

The National Fire Protection Association (NFPA) as well as the CGA has made recommendations related to safety in the use of cylinder gases. The first three recommendations listed below relate to the potential of fire hazard in oxygen-enriched environments.[5] This section will also cover some electrical and chemical hazards related to the potential for fire. (This description is not intended to cover electrical safety or the problems associated with drug administration.) Although oxygen is not explosive, substances that are combustible in air will burn rapidly in an oxygen-enriched atmosphere. In addition, substances that are normally not considered combustible, may burn in the presence of elevated oxygen levels.

A. Recommendations Concerning Fire Hazards

- *Combustible materials,* such as hair oils, aerosol sprays, oil-based lubricants (e.g., petroleum jelly), skin lotions, rubbing compounds or alcohol, and facial tissues, should be removed from the administration site. Mechanical pencils, pens, combs, toothbrushes, and some toys may be made of celluloid, which is extremely combustible even in air, should be removed from the room. Contamination of oxygen devices with oil or grease must be avoided, as they combine explosively under pressure. Flammable or combustible aerosols, such as alcohol and hair spray, must not be used in an oxygen-enriched atmosphere. Lubricants for beds and motors must be nonflammable. An ABC-type dry chemical fire extinguisher should be immediately available whenever home respiratory therapy is employed. In case of fire the following steps are recommended by the NFPA:[5]

1. If the patient is directly involved, it is of foremost importance to extinguish the flames, especially if the patient's hair or clothing is on fire.
2. Move the patient to safety.
3. Turn off the oxygen supply if this can be accomplished without personal danger. If the gas source can be moved with the patient, do so.
4. Close the doors to the room.
5. Notify the fire department.
6. Notify other occupants of the building.
7. If the fire is small and there is not a great deal of smoke present you may want to attempt to extinguish or contain the fire. However, if the fire is large or there is a significant amount of smoke present, leave the building and await the fire fighters. Oxygen-enriched atmospheres produce intensely hot fires.
8. Remain calm, think clearly, and act decisively.

- *Ignition* occurs much easier in an oxygen-enriched atmosphere, so all sources of ignition must be removed. No sources of open flame, including candles, heaters, or sparking toys, should be permitted in the room. Electrical equipment, even battery powered, can be a source of ignition in an oxygen-enriched environment. All electrical equipment should have a three-prong, grounded plug, or some other means of grounding the equipment should be provided. It is advisable to check three-prong outlets to assure that the ground connection is functional. Radios, televisions, remote-control devices, electric razors, electric toothbrushes, hair dryers, and reading lamps can be sources of ignition. Electrical appliances that get hot, that spark, or that smoke can ignite a fire, especially in an environment of an increased oxygen levels. Any electrical items suspected of being defective should be removed from the room and repaired. It should be noted that some respiratory therapy equipment is electrically powered and thus can also be an ignition source if defective, improperly grounded, or damaged in use. There may also be a serious shock hazard if respiratory therapy equipment is defective and generates leakage current, as gases containing aerosols and condensate can make the equipment conductive. Any electrical appliance that is not specifically approved for use in an oxygen-enriched environment should be kept at least 5 feet from the administration site. Opening the cylinder valve too quickly can generate heat from gas compression. Such heat production has been reported to have caused ignition and personal injury. Only solutions and medications prescribed by the patient's physician should be utilized in the administration devices. Static electricity does not have sufficient energy to be considered an ignition source under normal conditions, even in oxygen-enriched atmospheres, so long as easily ignited substances are not present. The NFPA does recommend that carpeting of wool and acrylic, nylon, and other synthetic fibers not be present in the area of administration unless the carpeting has been rendered permanently static proof.
- All *smoking materials* (matches, lighter, cigarettes, and tobacco) should be removed from the room. The patient and family must be instructed regarding the extreme dangers of smoking around respiratory therapy equipment, even if it is turned off. The family should also be

```
┌─────────────────────────────────────────────────┐
│                                                   │
│                   CAUTION                         │
│                                                   │
│               OXYGEN IN USE                       │
│                                                   │
│                NO SMOKING                         │
│                                                   │
│              NO OPEN FLAMES                       │
│                                                   │
├───────────────────────────────────────────────── │
│    Any material that can burn In alr will burn more rapidly In the │
│    presence of oxygen. No electrical equipment Is allowed within  an │
│         oxygen enclosure or within 5 ft. (1.5 m) of It.           │
└─────────────────────────────────────────────────┘
```

Figure 1.5 Minimum content for a no smoking precautionary sign.

instructed to alert visitors to these dangers. There should be at least one sign displayed in the room, readable from a distance of at least 5 feet. Figure 1.5 displays the minimum text for a precautionary "No Smoking" sign. Special signs should be used whenever foreign languages present a communication problem. It is advisable to post additional signs outside the doors leading into the room. Personal injury has been reported as a result of smoking or open flames near the site of oxygen administration.

B. Recommendations Concerning Mechanical Hazards

The recommendations covered in this section are those of the NFPA and CGA that relate to the storage and handling of cylinder gases, both in the home and at the home care company or facility.[5] Recommendations pertaining to other devices will be covered later.

- *Handling.* The careful handling of cylinders is necessitated by their weight as well as their pressurized contents. Large cylinders can weigh as much as 150 pounds and can cause crushing injury if dropped or tipped over. If the cylinder valve is damaged when a cylinder falls, the cylinder can become a missile with a 1-ton thrust.

- *Storage.* The cylinder storage area should afford protection from extreme cold and accumulations of ice and snow. The storage of cylinders outside or in unheated rooms can result in frostbite injury from contact with cold metal. Likewise, stored cylinders should not be subjected to extreme heat (temperatures exceeding 125 degrees F [52 degrees C]), nor should cold cylinders be warmed by heating. In storage, cylinders should be protected from tampering, cutting, and abrasion. The cylinder storage area should be permanently posted. The storage facility should be constructed of fire-resistant walls, where practical; should be free of flammable, highly combustible, and corrosive substances; and should be cool and dry, to prevent cylinder rusting. The facility should also be well ventilated, to prevent accumulation of oxygen in the event of a leak. Storing cylinders underground should be avoided, as should storing them in a closet or the trunk of a car. In the home, cylinders, whether full or empty, should be stored in accordance with the recommendations of the supplier. Large cylinders should be stored with their valves closed and their protective caps in place, and they must be secured to prevent tipping. Cylinders should be stored in groups according to contents, and gases that support combustion should be stored in a separate location from gases that are combustible. Full and empty cylinders should be separated.

- *Transport.* The patient and family should be educated in the proper handling of cylinders and carts during cylinder transport. A cart used to transport a large cylinder should be of self-supporting design, and the cylinder must be secured by a chain or strap. Cylinders should not be transported in the trunk of a car. If a cylinder is provided with a protective cap, it should be in place during transport and at all other times when the cylinder is not in use; however, the cylinder should not be lifted by the cap. Cylinders must not be allowed to drop, drag, slide, or strike together violently. Cylinders that are very cold should be handled with extreme care to prevent frostbite to bare skin. Cylinders should not come in contact with hands, gloves, or clothing contaminated with grease or oil.

- *Installation.* At the site of use, a cylinder must be secured by a chain or strap or otherwise supported by a cylinder base or cart that is designed not to tip over. A small cylinder should be attached to a cylinder stand or to a therapy apparatus of sufficient size to make the entire assembly stable; a cylinder must not be secured to the bed or other movable object. The cylinder must be positioned in such a way that it does not come in contact with a heat source or open flames. The cylinder labels must be clearly visible; must not be defaced, altered, or removed; and must *always* be checked before any gas is administered. The home care provider should assure that all safety suggestions and requirements have been considered in the design of delivery vehicles, carts, and other pertinent equipment.

- *Connection.* For the proper connection of a cylinder and the safe administration of gas, the following steps should be taken:

    1. After the cylinder has been secured (as described above) and the contents verified from the label, remove the protective cap and inspect the cylinder valve and apparatus to be sure they are free of foreign materials and oil.
    2. Turn the cylinder valve away from any people present , stand to the side, and quickly open and close the cylinder valve to remove any dust that might be present in the cylinder valve outlet. This will create noise, and it is advisable to warn occupants of the room of this fact ahead of time.
    3. Securely tighten, but never force, a pressure-reducing valve or regulator onto the cylinder valve outlet. Pressure-reducing valves must be used on high-pressure cylinders and should be listed for high-pressure service. Do not connect fixed or adjustable orifices or metering and other devices to a cylinder without a pressure-reducing valve or regulator. Place labels on pressure-reducing valves, regulators, and metering devices stating "OXYGEN—USE NO OIL" and stating gas for which the devices are intended, along with the name of the manufacturer or supplier. If calibration or function is dependent on gas density, device must be labeled as to the proper supply pressure.
    4. After making sure that the regulator or reducing valve is in the off or closed position, open the cylinder valve slowly to pressurize the reducing valve or regulator. Once pressurization has occurred, open the cylinder valve completely and then back one-fourth to one-half turn. Keep the cylinder valve closed at all times when it is not in use.
    5. When making connections, use wrenches that are free from oil and grease. Use only the appropriate wrenches supplied with the equipment. Do not use pipe wrenches.

```
CAUTION
OXYGEN IN USE
KEEP FLAMES AWAY
NO SMOKING
NO ELECTRICAL APPLIANCES
```

Figure 1.6 Minimum contact for an enclosure label.

6. Use only cylinder valve outlet connections that conform to ANSI B57.1 (American Standard and Pin Index Safety System) and low-pressure threaded connections that comply with the Diameter Index Safety System or are low-pressure quick connections of noninterchangeable design. Apparatus designed for one gas should not be used with another gas.

- *Operation, Repair and Maintenance*

1. Use only those service manuals, operator manuals, instructions, procedures, and repair parts provided or recommended by the manufacturer.
2. Allow only qualified personnel to service respiratory therapy equipment. Set aside a servicing area that is clean and free of oil and grease, that is designated for the servicing of oxygen equipment, and that is not used for the repair of other equipment.
3. Follow a scheduled preventive maintenance program.

C. Other Recommendations

- Humidifiers and nebulizers must be incapable of tipping or must be mounted in such a fashion that any tipping that can occur will not interfere with proper function or accuracy. Humidifiers and nebulizers must be equipped with an overpressure relief and/or alarm in the event of flow obstruction. Reservoir jars for humidifiers and nebulizers must be constructed of transparent materials to allow observation of the liquid level and must be impervious to solutions and medications used.

- Enclosures such as hoods and canopies should be labeled with warnings, the minimum recommended text of which is displayed in Figure 1.6. Labels should be placed in the interior of the enclosure in a position to be read by the patient and on two or more opposing sides of the exterior of the enclosure. Flexible canopies must be constructed of materials classified as "slow burning," and rigid enclosures must be fabricated of noncombustible material.

- The transfilling of cylinders is dangerous and should be done only at the site of the cylinder-gas supplier. The mixing of compressed gases in cylinders should never be done.

- Pressure in cylinders must be reduced to atmospheric pressure and evacuated to at least 25 inches of mercury vacuum prior to filling by the supplier. Only equipment provided by the manufacturer that complies with CGA Pamphlet P-2.5, "Transfilling of High Pressure Gaseous Oxygen To Be Used for Respiration," is to be utilized. The filling agency must affix labels to the cylinder as required by DOT or FDA regulations. The procedure used for filling cylinders must include adequate steps to assure the proper content of each cylinder, purity, color coding, labeling, and valving. Records must be kept to verify that these specifications have been met.

- Safety-relief devices, noninterchangeable quick connections, and other safety devices should not be removed, altered, or replaced.
- Devices should not be stored or transported with liquids in their reservoirs.
- Nasal catheters used in respiratory therapy should be green to prevent their accidental attachment to gastric or intestinal apparatus.
- Defective equipment must be removed from service immediately and serviced by qualified personnel only.
- *Cleaning/Sterilization*

1. High-pressure oxygen equipment must *not* be sterilized with substances containing flammable agents such as ethylene oxide or alcohol. Polyethylene, which may slough particles that are pure hydrocarbons and thus constitute a severe fire hazard, must not be used to package high-pressure oxygen equipment for sterilization.
2. A significant hazard is posed by residual sterilizing agent in respiratory therapy equipment.
3. Sterilizing agents must be oil free and must not be damaging to materials in the devices.
4. Respiratory therapy equipment operated at pressures below 60 pounds per square inch gauge may be sterilized with nonflammable mixtures containing ethylene oxide and carbon dioxide or fluorocarbon diluents.
5. Cylinders and oxygen containers must not be sterilized; generally it is sufficient for cylinders, and equipment attached directly to them, to be wiped off with a mild soap or disinfectant that is not damaging to plastic. The recommendations of the manufacturer or supplier should be followed.
6. Surface temperatures must not exceed 248 degrees F (120 degrees C) where diethyl ether is used, as it converts to formaldehyde upon contact with heating elements, such as those in an incubator.
7. Some gas mixtures may decompose when they come in contact with hot surfaces, producing toxic or flammable fumes or substances.

Estimating Duration of Gas Supply

Conversion factors for calculating how long a cylinder's contents will last are based upon Boyle's law, which states that the volume of gas varies inversely with its pressure. The amount of time that a cylinder will last depends on the size (or volume) of the cylinder, the pressure of its contents, and the flowrate at which gas is removed. The cylinder factor for each size cylinder is based on the cylinder content volume (in liters [L]) and filling pressure (in psig), as shown in the following examples:

$$\text{E cylinder factor} = \frac{622 \text{ L}}{2,200 \text{ psig}} = 0.3$$

$$\text{H cylinder factor} = \frac{6,600}{2,200 \text{ psig}} = 3.0$$

The cylinder factors for other sizes of cylinder can be calculated with the same formula if the cylinder contents volume is known. Sizes are frequently reported in cubic feet; multiplication of a cubic-foot value by 28.3 will yield the equivalent liter value.

The following formula can be used to estimate how long a cylinder's contents will last.

$$\frac{\text{Cylinder Pressure (psig)} \times \text{Cylinder Factor}}{\text{Flow Setting (L/min)}} = \text{Minutes}$$

For example, if a patient is going to use a full (2,200 psig) E cylinder at 2 L/min, the formula will yield an estimated contents duration of 5.5 hours, as shown below:

$$\frac{\text{Cylinder Pressure (psig)} \times \text{Cylinder Factor}}{\text{Flow Setting (L/min)}} = \text{Minutes}$$

$$\frac{2,200 \text{ psig} \times 0.3}{2 \text{ L/min}} = \frac{660}{2} = 330 \text{ Minutes, or 5.5 Hours}$$

The formula should be used only as an estimate, and the patient should be instructed to allow time in transit and never to let a cylinder approach empty.

Liquid-Oxygen Systems

In 1907 Dr. Karl von Linde accomplished fractional distillation of liquid air, which opened the way for bulk liquid-oxygen systems in hospitals and for smaller units in the home care.[1] Liquid oxygen expands about 860 times to become gaseous oxygen, so substantially less space is required to store the same amount of liquid oxygen as oxygen gas. This not only increases the supply and mobility capabilities for patients in the home but reduces the oxygen transportation costs, making it less expensive for the patient.

In the process of producing liquid oxygen, air is dried, filtered, and compressed to a pressure of about 200 atmospheres. The heat of compression is removed by running the compressed air through cooling coils. Once the compressed air is cooled, it is expanded to a pressure of 5 atmospheres, which drops the temperature of the compressed air to below -300 degrees F, and the gases in the air liquefy. Nitrogen and most of the other gases in air have a lower boiling point than that of oxygen, so they boil off (turn to gas) first as the liquid air is warmed. The nitrogen gas is drawn off, and the process is then repeated until the purity of the liquid oxygen is at least 99%. The liquid oxygen is then drawn off into reservoirs or transport tankers to be delivered to bulk reservoirs at supply or health care facilities.

Storage

The design of liquid-oxygen storage vessels is similar in principle to that of a thermos (Figure 1.7). The inner container, which holds the liquid and gaseous oxygen, is separated from the outer shell by insulation or a vacuum to block the transfer of heat. The liquid must be kept at a temperature of about -300 degrees F. This is accomplished by a pressure release mechanism. As the contents warm, the pressure rises until the release pressure is reached. When gas escapes through

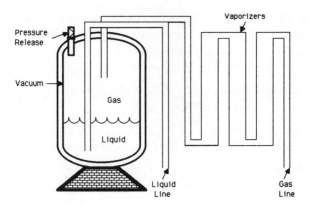

Figure 1.7 Bulk oxygen system.

the pressure release mechanism, more liquid oxygen expands to become gaseous oxygen, and this expansion cools the contents. As the contents cool, the pressure inside the container drops. Once the pressure is reduced below the release pressure, the release mechanism reseats and venting stops. This venting mechanism is present in all liquid-oxygen reservoirs, from the small units used in the home to the large bulk storage systems at the supplier's facility. Liquid can be siphoned off to fill other liquid vessels, or gas can be drawn off through vaporizing coils to fill cylinders.

Bulk Systems

Bulk storage of oxygen is defined as more than 20,000 cu. ft. of oxygen, including any unconnected reserves. Recommendations regarding the structure of bulk oxygen systems are made by the NFPA, the American Society of Mechanical Engineers (ASME), and the Bureau of Explosives (under regulations for pressure releases). The structure and installation of a bulk oxygen system should meet the NFPA specifications described below[6]:

- Bulk liquid oxygen vessels must be designed, tested, and constructed of materials that meet the impact-testing requirements of the ASME Boiler and Pressure Vessel Codes, section VII, and that are in accordance with DOT specifications and regulations for 4L liquid-oxygen containers. Insulation used in such containers must be of a noncombustible material. Containers for gas under high pressure must meet the design, testing, and construction requirements of the ASME Boiler and Pressure Vessel Code, section VIII. The vessel must be equipped with a safety-release device as required by the ASME Code, section IV, and and the provisions of ASME S-1.3 or DOT regulations and specifications for both the container and safety releases. The insulation casings must be equipped with suitable safety-release devices designed and located so that moisture cannot freeze or otherwise interfere with proper operation. Vaporizing columns and connection piping must be anchored in a manner to be sufficiently flexible for the expansion and contraction that results from temperature changes. The vaporizer and piping should be protected with safety-relief devices. If heat is supplied to the vaporizers, it must be done in an indirect fashion, such as with steam, air, water, or water-based solutions that do not react with oxygen, and the vaporizer is to be grounded if liquid heaters are used. Joints in the piping connections should be welded, flanged, threaded-slip, or compressed fittings. All gaskets, threaded seals, valves, gauges, and regulators placed into the system must be designed for oxygen service. Piping must conform to ANSI B31.3 and piping that operates below -20 degrees F must be composed of materials meeting ASME Code, section VIII. Containers, valves, gauges, and regulators must be protected from physical damage and tampering. Any enclosure containing control equipment must be adequately ventilated.

- The permanent installation of liquid-oxygen systems must be supervised by personnel familiar with proper installation and construction as outlined in NFPA 50. The bulk oxygen system must be mounted on supports and foundations that are noncombustible. A surface of noncombustible material must be provided that extends at least 3 feet beyond points where leakage of liquid oxygen could occur during system operation or filling. Asphalt or bitumastic paving is prohibited, and the slope of an area must be considered in the sizing of the surface. The same type of surface must extend at least the full width of the vehicle that fills the bulk unit and at least 8 feet in the transverse direction. Weeds and tall grass must be kept back 15 feet from the oxygen container. No part of the system should be underneath electrical power lines or within the reach of a downed power line, nor should any part of the system be exposed to flammable gases or to piping containing any class of flammable or combustible liquids. All components of the system are to be cleaned prior to being placed into service, so that oxidizable substances are removed, and all field-erected piping must be tested for leaks at maximum operating pressure with an oil-free, nonflammable gas medium. The site of the liquid-oxygen vessel is to be permanently posted **"OXYGEN—NO SMOKING—NO OPEN FLAMES."** The location of the system must be readily accessible to mobile supply equipment at ground level and to authorized personnel. The system must be inspected regularly by a qualified representative of the liquid-oxygen supplier. Figure 1.8 displays the minimum distance requirements for a bulk oxygen system as they relate to an oxygen supplier. A complete listing for health care facilities can be found in NFPA No. 50, Bulk Oxygen Systems.

Home Systems

Smaller versions of the bulk storage systems provide home liquid-oxygen units. A main supply unit (Figure 1.9), which provides the liquid-oxygen source, is basically a miniature version of the larger systems, with a vacuum or other insulation between the inner and outer containers. Liquid can be siphoned off to fill a smaller, portable device, or gas can flow through the vaporizer coils to supply the patient with oxygen in the home. A carrier for portable liquid air units is available from Air Lift (Figure 1.10). The portable device is designed to supply only gaseous oxygen via its vaporizer coil. Most liquid-oxygen devices designed for the home keep the contents at a pressure of about 20 psig with the use of a venting mechanism as described above. The Linde devices are an exception as they keep the contents pressure at about 90 psig. Oxygen flow is controlled by set-sized orifices or flow-restrictors that are calibrated at 20 psig or some other supply pressure value.

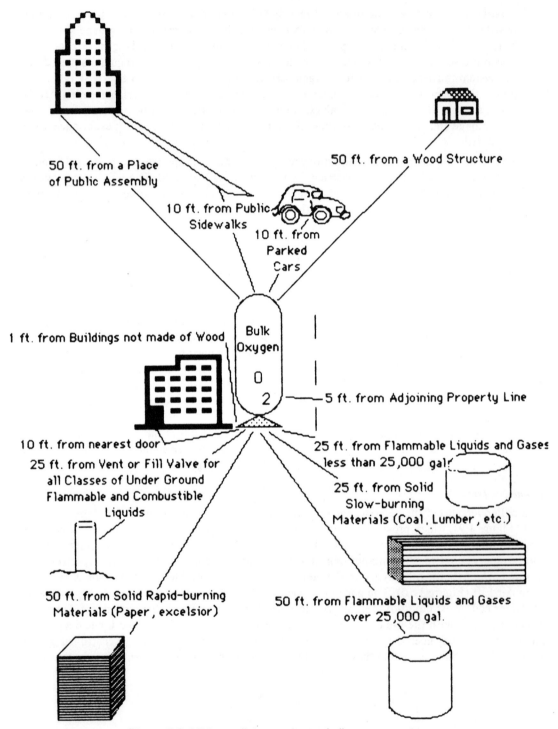

Figure 1.8 Minimum distances from a bulk oxygen system.

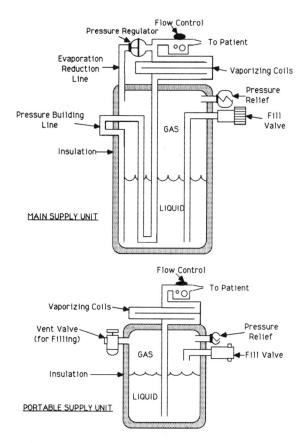

Figure 1.9 Liquid oxygen units for the home are smaller versions of bulk oxygen supply systems.

Devices that cause significant back pressure should not be attached, as they will alter the pressure gradient necessary for gas to flow through the orifice of the flow control, and the set flow will not be delivered. When checking home liquid-oxygen devices, one should inspect the fill valves and vents for damage or wear and verify the set flow from the device with a Thorpe tube flow tester. Table 1.1 lists common liquid oxygen devices and their specifications.

Most liquid-oxygen systems deliver oxygen continuously at the flow set on the device. The $Cryo_2$ Pulsair I and II have the capability of delivering oxygen on inspiration only through a demand valve that senses inspiration. Limited published reports have indicated that the pulse delivery of oxygen from a liquid device can reduce the consumption of oxygen by as much as 67%.[7]

Estimating Duration of Gas Supply

Liquid-oxygen devices increase both the amount of oxygen that can be stored in the home and the amount that can be transported in the portable device. Calculation of how long liquid oxygen will last is not based on the contents pressure, as with cylinder gas, but rather on the weight of

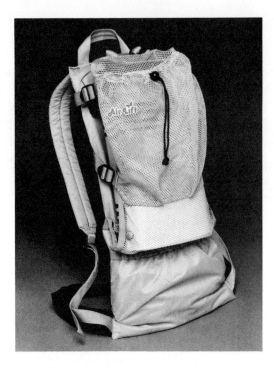

Figure 1.10 Carrier for portable liquid units.
Courtesy of AirLift.

the liquid. As mentioned earlier, liquid oxygen expands about 860 times to become gas. If the gas capacity of the reservoir is known, a simple calculation of the gauge reading multiplied times the capacity will provide the amount of gas supply left. If this figure is divided by the flow setting, the time that the liquid contents will last is calculated in minutes.

$$\text{Contents Remaining} = \text{Capacity} \times \text{Gauge Reading}$$

As an example, if the device's capacity is 1,000 liters and the gauge reads 3/4 full, the remaining capacity can be calculated.

$$\text{Contents Remaining} = \text{Capacity} \times \text{Gauge Reading}$$
$$\text{Contents Remaining} = 1{,}000 \text{ liters} \times 3/4$$
$$\text{Contents Remaining} = \frac{3{,}000}{4} = 750 \text{ liters}$$

If the patient is using the device at a flow of 1 liter per minute, the duration of the contents can be calculated as follows:

$$\text{Duration of Contents} = \frac{\text{Contents Remaining}}{\text{Flow}}$$
$$\text{Duration of Contents} = \frac{750 \text{ liters}}{1 \text{ L/min}} = 750 \text{ minutes, or 12 hrs. and 30 min.}$$

In small liquid containers, there is generally a gauge that displays the level or weight of the liquid remaining. Liquid oxygen weighs 2.5 pounds per liter, so the amount in liters of liquid oxygen can be calculated by simply dividing the weight of the contents by 2.5. If the weight of the contents is not displayed, it can be computed by weighing the vessel and its contents and subtracting the weight of the container when empty. Once the weight of the contents is determined, it is divided by 2.5.

Because a liquid liter of oxygen expands to become 860 gaseous liters, the gas-supply duration can be estimated from the weight of the remaining liquid.

$$\text{Gas Supply Remaining} = \frac{\text{Liquid Weight} \times 860}{2.5 \text{ lb}}$$

If the liquid weight is 3 pounds, and the patient is planning to use the gas contents at 1.5 liters per minute, the calculations will be as follows:

$$\text{Gas Supply Remaining} = \frac{\text{Liquid Weight} \times 860}{2.5 \text{ lb}}$$

$$\text{Gas Supply Remaining} = \frac{3 \text{ lbs} \times 860}{2.5 \text{ lb}} = \frac{2{,}580}{2.5} = 1{,}032 \text{ liters}$$

$$\text{Duration of Contents} = \frac{\text{Gas Supply Remaining}}{\text{Flow}}$$

$$\text{Duration of Contents} = \frac{1{,}032 \text{ liters}}{1.5 \text{ L/min}} = 688 \text{ minutes, or 11 hrs and 28 min}$$

Safety Recommendations

The NFPA recommendations for cylinders, described in an earlier section, also apply to liquid-oxygen devices. In addition, the following are safety recommendations specific to home liquid-oxygen units:[5]

- When liquid-oxygen devices are not in use, oxygen will vent (as described earlier) and can create an oxygen-enriched environment, especially if the device is stored in a closed space. Larger than normal amounts of oxygen will be vented if the container is accidentally tipped over or placed on its side. Devices containing liquid oxygen should be stored in well-ventilated areas to prevent the creation of an oxygen-enriched atmosphere. The transfer of liquid oxygen from one container to another may create an elevated oxygen atmosphere. Liquid-oxygen devices should never be stored in closets or transported in the trunk of a car, nor should they be placed in the proximity of radiators, steam pipes, or heat ducts. Liquid-oxygen containers should not be handled with hands, gloves, or clothing contaminated with oil or grease. The contents of the containers should be verified by personnel when setting up the equipment and when changing the containers. Connections for containers are to be made in accordance with the container manufacturer's operating instructions. The patient and family must be familiar with the proper operation of the liquid-oxygen devices and be instructed as to all precautions and safeguards.

- Frostbite can occur if liquid-oxygen devices are tipped over and the liquid oxygen comes in contact with the skin. Similar injury can occur during the transfer of liquid from one container to another if the connections are improperly made or a malfunction occurs. The transfer

Table 1.1 Specifications for Liquid Oxygen Units

Liquid Units	Liquid Capacity (L)	Gas Equivalent Liters NTP	Operating Pressure PSIG	Flow Rates Available LPM	Dimensions H W inches		Diameter inches	Empty Weight lbs.	Full Weight lbs.	Evap. Rates (lbs/day)
CRYO$_2$ Corp.										
Grandeair II	37.0 L	31,908	20	0–8	31.3" H		16.0 D	47	140	1.5
Stationair II	25.5 L	21,033	20	0–8	25.5" H		16.0 D	37	99	1.3
Travelair I	1.08 L	865	20	0,1,1.5,2, 2.5,3,4,5	H 1.35" ×	W 8.2"	5.5 D	7.0	9.5	1.3
Travelair II	1.81 L	1,560	20	0,1,1.5,2, 2.5,3,4,5	H 14.5 ×	W 10.1	6.9 D	9.3	13.8	1.5
Wanderair II-D	0.49 L	400	20	0,1,1.5,2 2.5,3,4,5	H 10.4 ×	W 7.2	5.0 D	5.3	6.5	1.3
Pulsair I	0.49 L	400	20	0,1,1.5,2, 2.5,3,4,5	H 10.4 ×	W 7.2	5.0 D	5.9	7.1	1.3
Pulsair II	1.08L	865	20	0,1,1.5,2, 2.5,3,4,5	H 13.5 ×	W 8.2	5.5 D	7.6	10.1	1.3
Cryogenic Assoc.										
Stroller Sprint	.60 L	513	20	.25,.5,.75, 1,1.5,2,3	H 10.5		oval	5.4	6.9	1.0
Stroller	1.23 L	1,058	20	.25,.5,.75,1, 1.5,2,2.5, 3,4,6 (no.5)	H 13.5		oval	6.5	9.5	1.0
Liberator 20	20 L	17,200	20	.25,.5,.75, 1,1.5,2,2.5 3,4,6 (no.5)	H 27.8		12.0 D	35.0	85.0	1.0

Liberator 30	30 L	25,800	20	.25,.5,.75 1,1.5,2,2.5 3,4,6 (no. 5)	H 35.0	12.0 D	46.5	120.0	1.0
Liberator 45	42.0 L	36,120	20	.25,.5,.75 1,1.5,2,2.5 3,4,6 (no. 5)	H 35.0	14.0 D	57.0	163.0	1.8
Mt. Med. Equip., Inc.									
Escort Base Reservoir #302.005.801	28.0 L	24,097	22	—	—	—	43.0	116.0	1.1
Escort Base Reservoir #302.005.803	40.0 L	34,186	22	—	—	—	51.0	151.0	1.1
Escort Portable Low Flow #302.005.807	0.5 L	430	21	0–8	—	—	5.5	6.5	1.1
Escort Port. Standard #302.005.805	1.0 L	860	21	0–8	—	—	6.25	8.5	1.1
Escort Port. Standard #302.005.806	2.0 L	1,721	21	0–8	—	—	7.5	12.0	1.1
Penox Tech., Inc.									
Mini Base Unit	18. L	15,480	—	0–8 ped. avail.	H 23.0	D 18.0	38	89	—
Standard Base Unit	28. L	24,097	—	0–8 ped. avail.	H 27.0	D 18.0	43	116.0	—

Table 1.1—*Continued*

Liquid Units	Liquid Capacity (L)	Gas Equivalent Liters NTP	Operating Pressure PSIG	Flow Rates Available LPM	Dimensions H W inches	Diameter inches	Empty Weight lbs.	Full Weight lbs.	Evap. Rates (lbs/day)
Large Base Unit	40.0 L	34,186	—	0–8 ped. avail.	H 33.0	D 18.0	51	151	—
Penox Portable I	0.5 L	430	—	1,1.5,2, 2.5,3,4,5 ped. avail. HF (1–8) avail.	H 10.75	D 7. × 6.	5.5	6.5	—
Penox Port. II	1.0 L	860	—	1,1.5,2,2.5, 3,4,5 ped. avail. HF (1–8) avail.	H 13.0	D 7. × 6.5	6.25	8.5	—
Penox Port. III	2.0 L	1,721	—	1,1.5,2,2.5 3,4,5 ped. avail. HF (1–8) avail.	H 13.75	D 7. × 6.5	7.5	12	—
Puritan Bennett									
Companion T 775532	1.23 L	1,058	22	up to 15 LPM	H 14.4	—	5.3	8.5	—
Companion T5 775510	31 L	25,523	19.5	up to 15 LPM	H 32.0	D 14.25	75	125	—
Union Carbide									
UCC Mark III OR.302 Small Cylinder	16 L	13,800	50	12 LPM Max	H 25	D 15 3/16"	27.	70 approx.	1.5

UCC Mark III OR.303 Large Cylinder	28 L	24,100	50	12 LPM Max	H 32.6	D 13.3	38.	110 approx.	1.3
UCC Mark III Walker OW.303	.64 L	550	50	1–5	H × W 11 × 9.3	D 5.3	5 w/o strap	6.6 w/o strap	1.0
UCC Mark III Walker OW.302	1.27 L	1,092	50	1–5	H × W 13.5 × 9.4	D 5.6	8.3	11.5	1.0
Puritan Bennett									
Companion 31	31 L	25,523	19.5	6 LPM Max	H 32	D 14.25	51	130 approx.	1.8
Companion 1000	1.23 L	1,058	21	1,1.5,2,2.5 3,4,6 (no.5)	H 13.4″	contoured	4.5	7.6	1.5

of liquid oxygen from one container to another for use in the home is to be done using equipment designed to comply with the performance requirements of CGA Pamphlet P-2.6, "Transfilling of Low Pressure Liquid Oxygen To Be Used for Respiration," and in accordance with the manufacturer's operating instructions. All liquid containers must meet DOT 4L specifications (all connections used must comply with ANSI B57.1 P CSA B96, or the manufacturer's non-interchangeable liquid-oxygen connections). All containers must have a pressure release to limit the container pressure to specification pressure, and a device must be used to limit the amount of liquid oxygen introduced into the container to the manufacturer's rated capacity. All connections used in filling must conform to CGA V-1, and the hose assembly must have a pressure release set no higher than the container's rated pressure. Transfilling of liquid containers must be performed in a well ventilated area. Delivery vehicles should be vented to prevent the buildup of high oxygen levels, and transfilling should occur with the delivery vehicle doors wide open. No smoking signs must be posted, and no sources of ignition can exist within five feet. Only filling equipment supplied by the manufacturer that comply with CGA Pamphlet P-2.6 is to be used. The transfiller must affix labels as required by DOT and FDA regulations. Records and instructions must state the proper content, purity, color coding, and labeling. All devices must be moisture free to prevent freezing, and pressure releases must function and be positioned correctly to prevent buildup of high pressures.

When liquid oxygen is spilled, the liquid tends to cover the entire suface and thus cools a large area. The gas escaping from the area is also very cold and can cause frostbite and injury to the eyes. Safety goggles with side shields should be worn, along with loose-fitting, properly insulated gloves, when liquid oxygen is handled. High-top boots, with cuffless pants worn outside of the boots, are also recommended.[8] Items that have been exposed to liquid oxygen should not be touched; in addition to causing frostbite, the objects can stick to skin. Materials that are pliable or soft at room temperature become brittle at the cold temperatures of liquid oxygen. If liquid oxygen is spilled, the cold liquid and resulting gas condense the moisture in the air, creating a fog that except in extremely dry climates normally extends over an area that is larger than the area of contact danger.[8] As mentioned previously, liquid oxygen spilled on asphalt or oil-soaked concrete constitutes an extreme hazard, and an explosive reaction can occur. If a spill does occur, measures should be taken to prevent anyone from walking on the surface or wheeling any equipment over the area of the spill, and all sources of ignition should be kept away for at least 15 minutes or until all frost has disappeared.[9] If liquid oxygen or the resulting gas comes in contact with a person's skin, any clothing that may constrict blood flow to the frozen area should be removed and the affected area(s) warmed with water that is near body temperature.[8] If there is blistering of the skin or a chance that the eyes were affected, treatment by a physician should be sought immediately. Any clothing that has been contaminated with liquid oxygen should be removed and aired away from sources of ignition for at least an hour to be completely freed of oxygen.[9]

Piping Systems

The purpose of piping gases into the home from a central supply point is to make therapy more convenient and to increase patient mobility. When a gas-piping system is used, it must comply with the standards of NFPA 56F, specifically those outlined for nonhospital facilities whose storage capacity is not more than 2,000 cubic feet of gaseous oxygen or 5,000 cubic feet in DOT 4L liquid containers.[10] A home gas source can be of three types.

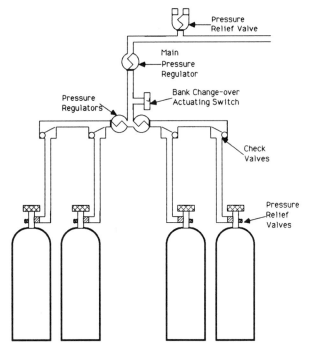

Figure 1.11 Alternating manifold oxygen supply system.

Alternating Manifold System

The first type of home gas source is the *alternating manifold system* (Figure 1.11), and is the most common type installed when cylinders are used as the gas source. All cylinders in a supply system must be designed, constructed, tested, and maintained according to DOT specifications and regulations. The cylinder manifold must have two banks that alternately supply the piping system. Each bank of the manifold must have a pressure regulator, and cylinders must be connected to a common header. Each bank must contain a minimum of two cylinders and at least an average day's supply of oxygen. When one bank is depleted to the point that it cannot supply the system, the other bank must automatically supply the system, and an activating switch should be connected to the master signal panel to indicate the changeover. A check valve is required for each cylinder lead and each manifold header to prevent the loss of gas from the entire bank or system if a pressure release on any individual cylinder should fail.

Alternating Manifold System with a Reserve Supply

The second type of cylinder system is similar to the first type except that it has a reserve supply (Figure 1.12) . This type of system, composed of the alternating manifold (primary and secondary supplies) and a reserve supply, operates in the same manner as the system described above, but its *reserve supply* operates automatically in the event that both the primary and secondary supplies become exhausted. The reserve supply must contain three or more cylinders that constitute at least an average day's supply of oxygen, and they must be connected to the system in the same

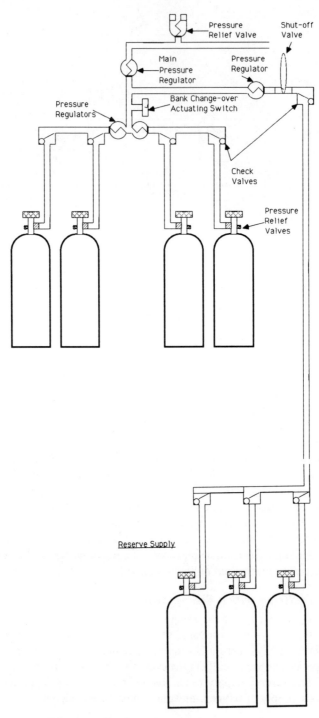

Figure 1.12 Alternating supply system with a reserve supply.

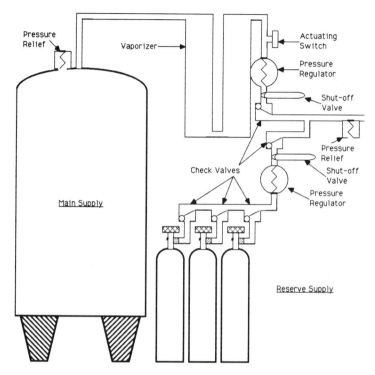

Figure 1.13 Continuous supply system with a reserve supply.

manner described above for manifolds. An activating switch must be connected to the master panel to indicate when the system is on the reserve supply. Another switch must be activated when the reserve drops to the one-day-supply level. If a liquid-oxygen system is installed, it must be installed with a reserve supply.

Continuous-Supply System with a Reserve Supply

The third type of supply system has one main source that continually supplies the piping system and a reserve supply, not normally in operation, that supplies the system only in an emergency (Figure 1.13). This type of system is usually employed when liquid oxygen is the main source and when the main supply is refilled on a frequent basis. If a liquid-oxygen device is used as the reserve, it must be provided with a switch that will activate an alarm if the gas pressure drops below the level required to supply the system in the event of loss of the main supply. If a liquid-oxygen device is designed to prevent loss of gas through evaporation, the gas must pass through the line pressure regulator before entering the piping system.

Safety Recommendations

The design of piping systems incorporates, and their specifications outline, safety features to protect them. If the liquid-oxygen containers are designed to prevent the loss of vented gas from the container, the vented gas must pass through the line pressure regulator before entering the piping system. The liquid-oxygen containers themselves must be constructed to withstand pressures of 2,200 psig or must be provided with suitable pressure-relief devices. If gas cylinders are used as the source in a system that contains primary, secondary, and reserve supplies, check valves are not required for each cylinder lead. Manifolds are to be designed and constructed of materials suitable for the gases and pressures involved. Cylinder valve outlets must comply with the American Canadian Standard for connections, a mechanical means of assuring the connection of the proper gas. The piping system must be capable of delivering oxygen at 50–55 psig to all outlets at maximum flowrate. A pressure regulator must be installed in the main supply line upstream from the final line-pressure-relief valve, and a manual shutoff valve must be installed upstream from each pressure regulator and shutoff valve (or a check valve must be installed downstream). The system must have a pressure-relief valve, set at 50% above normal line pressure, installed downstream from the pressure regulator and upstream from the shutoff valve. All pressure-relief valves must be of the type that close automatically when excess pressure has been released and should be vented to the outside if the supply system is in excess of 2,000 cu. ft. of gas. The pressure relief-valves are to be made of brass or bronze and designed for use with the specific gas service. Supply systems with a reserve supply must have a check valve in the main supply line upstream from the connecting points of the secondary and reserve supplies.

Medical Air Systems

If a *medical air* system is installed, it must draw its source of air from the outside atmosphere and should not draw in contaminants such as particulate matter, odor, or other gases. The air-intake port must be located where no contamination from engine exhausts, fuel storage vents, vacuum system discharges, or other particulate matter or odor of any type can be anticipated. A maintenance program following the manufacturer's recommendations is to be established. Air-intake ports must be located outdoors, above roof level, at a minimum of 20 feet above the ground, and at a minimum distance of 10 feet from any door, window or other intake or opening in the building, Intake ports must be turned downward and screened. At least two or more oil-free air compressors must be duplexed together, with provisions for operation alternately or simultaneously depending on demand. The compressor must be capable of maintaining the air supply to the system at calculated peak demand. An automatic means of preventing backflow through units that are off-cycled must be provided. Each duplex system should be provided with disconnect switches; with motor starting devices (with overload protection); with a means of automatic alternation of the compressors, with usage divided evenly, and with an automatic means of activating the additional compressor(s) in the event that the unit that is the source of supply becomes incapable of maintaining adequate pressure. The air storage tank (receiver) must have a safety valve, automatic drain, pressure gauge, and the capacity to ensure practical on-off operation. The type of medical air compressor and local atmospheric conditions will govern the provision of intake filter-mufflers (dry type), aftercoolers for air dryers, and additional downstream pressure regulators. Antivibration mountings, in accordance with manufacturer's recommendations, are to be installed under components and flexible couplings that connect air compressors, receiver, intake lines, and supply line.

Supply-System Location

The location of the supply system must be outside or in a building, enclosure, or room in a building that is used for this purpose only. Medical air and vacuum pumps must be in a separate location from that of the cylinder gas system. The walls, floors, ceiling, doors, interior finish, shelves, racks, and supports of the site must be constructed of materials that are noncombustible or of limited combustibility. For a system of more than 2,000 cubic-foot capacity, the walls, floors, and ceilings of the site that separate the system from other rooms in the building must have a fire resistance rating of at least one hour. Doors to the site must have louvered openings of at least 72 square inches. Sites for systems of more than 2,000 cubic feet must be vented to the outside. Doors or gates into the supply site must be locked. Regular electrical wall fixtures must be installed at least 5 feet above the floor to avoid physical damage. If the supply system is located near sources of heat, such as furnaces, incinerators, or boilers, the cylinders must be protected from reaching temperatures exceeding 130 degrees F. Open electrical conductors and transformers should not be located in close proximity to the system's site. Smoking is prohibited. Heating of the room must be by steam, hot water, or other indirect means, and the temperature must not exceed 130 degrees F. If the oxygen supply is located outside the building, an inlet for connecting a temporary auxiliary source of supply must be incorporated for emergency and maintenance situations. The inlet must be physically protected to prevent tampering or unauthorized access and should be labeled **Emergency Low-Pressure Gaseous Oxygen Inlet.** The inlet is to be installed downstream from the shutoff valve on the main supply line and should have the necessary valves to provide the emergency supply of oxygen plus the isolation of the pipeline to the normal source of supply. There must be a check valve in the main line between the inlet connection and the main shutoff valve and another check valve between the inlet connection and the emergency supply shutoff valve. The inlet connection must have a pressure-relief valve of adequate size to protect downstream piping from pressure in excess of 50% above normal pipeline pressure.

Supply-System Alarms

Warning and alarm systems are required to monitor the operation and condition of the supply system. Alarms and gauges are to be located so that the best possible surveillance can be made. Each alarm and gauge must be appropriately labeled. The master alarm system must monitor the source of supply, the reserve (if present), and the main line pressure of the gas system. The power source for warning systems must meet the essentials of NFPA 76A. All alarms must be evaluated and the necessary measures taken to reestablish or ensure the proper function of the supply system. Two master alarm panels, with noncancellable alarms, are to be located in separate locations to assure continuous observation. One signal is to be provided that will alert the user to a changeover from one operating supply to another, and an additional signal will provide notification that the reserve is supplying the system. If check valves are not installed in the cylinder leads and headers, another alarm signal should be initiated when the reserve reaches a one day's supply of oxygen. All piping systems must have an audible and a noncancellable visual signal to indicate when the main line pressure increases or decreases 20% from normal supply pressure. A pressure gauge must be installed and appropriately labeled adjacent to the switch that generates the over- or under-pressure alarm. All warning systems must be tested before being placed in service or being added to existing service, and periodic retesting and test records are required.

Piping-System Construction and Assembly

The construction and assembly of the piping system must also meet specifications. Piping must be of seamless type K or L copper tubing or standard weight brass pipe. The pipe size must be in conformity with good engineering practices and must provide the proper flows specified. Piping must be supported by pipe hooks, metal straps, bands, or hangers that are suitable for the pipe size and placed at proper intervals. Gas piping must not be supported by other piping. The fittings used for connecting copper tubing must be of wrought copper, brass, or bronze and made especially for solder or brazed connections. Brass pipe must be assembled with screw-type brass fittings or with bronze or copper brazing fittings. Buried piping must be adequately protected against frost, corrosion, and physical damage. Ducts or casings must be used whenever buried piping traverses a roadway, driveway, parking lot, or other area subject to surface loads. Piping in a combustible partition must be protected against physical damage by being installed within pipe or conduit. Openings for piping installed in concealed spaces must be fire-stopped with material having a fire resistance equal to or greater than the original construction. If the installation of medical gas piping in a kitchen, laundry, or other area of special hazard is unavoidable, the piping must be placed in an enclosure that will prevent the gas from entering the room should leaks occur. Piping exposed to physical damage must be suitably protected. The gas content of medical gas piping must be identified by appropriate labeling at least every 20 feet and at least once in every room. Piping must not be used as a grounding electrode.

Before installation, the piping, valves, and fittings must be thoroughly cleaned of oil, grease, and other readily oxidizable materials (except those especially prepared for oxygen service by the manufacturer and received sealed). The washing of nonsealed piping, valves, and fittings is accomplished by using a hot solution of sodium carbonate or trisodium phosphate. **(The use of organic solvents, such as CARBON TETRACHLORIDE, is *PROHIBITED*.)** The use of flux is prohibited in all instances except those requiring the joining of copper and brass or other dissimilar metals. When flux is used, particular care must be used in application to avoid leaving excess flux inside the completed joints. A visual inspection of each joint is required, and all hardened flux must be removed so that it does not cause a temporary seal. The outside of all tubes, joints, and fittings must be cleaned by hot-water washing after assembly. Threaded joints must be tinned or made with polytetrafluoroethylene tape or other thread sealants suitable for oxygen service. Sealants are to be applied to the male threads only. Following the installation of the piping and before the installation of the station outlets and other system components, the line is to be blown clear by means of oil-free, dry air or nitrogen.

Shutoff valves that are accessible must be installed in valve boxes that have breakable or removable windows and that are large enough to permit the operation of the valves, and the boxes must be labeled "CAUTION—[Name of the Medical Gas] VALVE: DO NOT CLOSE EXCEPT IN EMERGENCY. This Valve Controls Supply To. . . ." The main supply line shutoff valve is to be located where it is accessible in an emergency. If risers are installed to supply other floors of the home, a shutoff valve must be provided adjacent to the riser connection. Each branch of the supply line must have a shutoff valve, and no outlet should be supplied directly from a branch where the shutoff valve is located on another floor. Shutoff valves and additions to existing systems must be tested to verify proper operation and areas of control before being used.

Station outlets, whether of the threaded, DISS, or noninterchangeable quick-connect type, must be specific for the gas used and must have at least a primary and a secondary valve assembly. The secondary valve must close automatically to stop the flow of gas when the primary valve is removed. Each outlet must be labeled with the name or chemical symbol of the gas contained. Station outlets must be located at an appropriate height above the floor and must be recessed or otherwise protected to prevent physical damage to the outlet and attached equipment. When multiple wall outlets are installed, there must be sufficient spacing to permit the simultaneous use of adjacent outlets. Pressure gauges and manometers for medical gas piping must be cleaned, degreased, and identified: **[Name of Gas]—USE NO OIL!**

Piping-System Testing

After assembly of the piping system, a series of pressure tests is required to assure that the system is leak free and to be sure that no lines have been crossed. After installation of the station outlets but before the attachment of alarms and other components and before the walls are closed, each section of pipe is to be submitted to a minimum test pressure of 150 psig with oil-free, dry air or nitrogen. The test pressure is to be maintained until each joint has been examined for leakage by means of soapy water or another equally effective means of leak detection that is safe for use with oxygen. If a leak is found in any of the joints, the joint must be repaired and retested. Following the attachment of alarms and other components, the system must be subjected to a 24-hour static pressure test with oil-free, dry air or nitrogen at a pressure 20% above normal operating pressure. After the system is pressurized to the test level, the test gas is removed, and the system must remain leak free for 24 hours. Only those pressure changes caused by fluctuations in temperature are allowed. If any leaks are found, they must be repaired and the system retested. Prior to the connection of any extension or addition to the piping system, all tests mentioned must be performed, and records kept verifying the results. The final connection between any additions and the existing system must then be examined at normal operating pressure with soapy water or another effective means that is safe for use with oxygen. To determine that no cross-connections between systems exist, all systems are reduced to atmosphere and each system is pressurized independent of the others. With one system pressurized, all outlets of all systems are checked to verify that they are connected properly and that the test gas is being dispensed only from the outlets of the gas system being tested. That system is then reduced to atmospheric pressure, another is pressurized, and the same procedure is completed. This process continues until all systems have been checked. After all medical gas systems have been tested in this manner, the proper source of gas supply is connected to each system and pressurization occurs. All outlets must be opened in order, beginning with the outlet nearest the source and continuing through the system to the outlet farthest from the source. The gas purging the system should be allowed to pass through a white cloth material at a minimum flowrate of 100 L/min until no evidence of discoloration or odor is evident. After purging is complete, the gas from each station outlet for oxygen, medical air, and mixed gases containing oxygen must be tested with an oxygen analyzer to confirm the desired oxygen percentage.

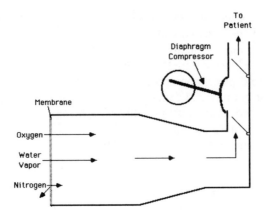

Figure 1.14 Membrane-type oxygen concentrator.

Oxygen Concentrators

Oxygen concentrators use a medium through which oxygen passes more easily than nitrogen. There are two basic types of oxygen concentrators.

The first type of oxygen concentrator employs a *thin membrane* that is about one micron (1/25,000th of an inch) thick. A diaphragm-type compressor creates a constant vacuum and draws gas across the membrane (Figure 1.14). Oxygen and water vapor are more permeable than is nitrogen, and the resulting gas passing through the membrane is concentrated with oxygen. Because nitrogen does not pass through the membrane as easily, the gas flowing from the other side of the membrane, through the flowmeter to the patient, is approximately 40% oxygen. Higher flows of gas to the patient's cannula are required to achieve the same blood gas levels as those achieved with a 100% oxygen source. This type of concentrator is produced by the Oxygen Enrichment, Ltd.

The second type of oxygen concentrator, by far the more common, uses a *molecular sieve* to remove nitrogen from the air. A compressor pumps room air to the sodium-aluminum silicate pellets that comprise the sieve beds (Figure 1.15). Oxygen (along with argon) passes freely through the sieve beds, while nitrogen, carbon dioxide, carbon monoxide, water vapor, and hydrocarbons are trapped. The resulting gas leaving the sieve beds of the concentrator is in excess of 90% oxygen; the gas flows to a reservoir, then to a flowmeter and on to the patient. Concentrators have been shown to be significantly unaffected by altitude.[11] Because the sieve beds trap nitrogen, they should be periodically purged. This is done by causing one sieve bed to receive a backflow to remove the nitrogen while the other sieve bed supplies oxygen to the patient; the process is then reversed, and the other sieve bed is purged. Table 1.2 gives specifications for some common brands of oxygen concentrators.

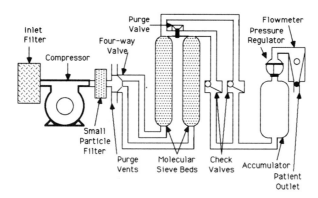

Figure 1.15 Molecular-sieve oxygen concentrator.

Oxygen concentrators should not be supplied with tubing lengths that exceed 50 feet unless the manufacturer is consulted. Placement of the concentrator in the home must not impede air from being freely drawn in through the air-intake ports, and the concentrator must not be placed near sources of heat. When checking a concentrator in the home, one should verify both the oxygen percentage being delivered and the flow being supplied; the percentage delivered can be checked with an oxygen analyzer, and the flow can be checked with a Thorpe tube flow measuring device. All filters, along with alarms, batteries, etc., should be checked in accordance with following the manufacturers' recommendations. Because oxygen concentrators are electrically powered, a reserve source of oxygen must be present in the event of a power failure. The patient and family must be instructed in all aspects of safety and proper care of the concentrator.

Air Compressors

Air compressors provide an air source to power other devices used in respiratory home care. Small compressors are used to power medication nebulizers, larger volume nebulizers, oxygen concentrators, and some intermittent positive pressure breathing (IPPB) devices. Larger compressors with a compressed air reservoir, can be used to supply compressed air to mechanical ventilators.

Three basic types of compressors used in respiratory home care (Figure 1.16). The first type is the *piston-type compressor* in which the motor drives the piston and rod up and down. The downward motion of the piston draws gas into the cylinder through the intake valve; and as the piston moves upward, the intake valve is closed and air is forced out of the exhaust valve. Various types of materials are used for the rings that seal the piston against the cylinder wall. An outflow filter is preferable, especially with carbon ring compressors, to trap any flakes that occur as the rings wear. *Lubrication with oil must be avoided.* Piston compressors are generally used when

Table 1.2 Specifications for Oxygen Concentrators

	Manufactures Specifications for Percentage 1L/M	2L/M	3L/M	4L/M	5L/M	6L/M	Flow Control Type	Delivery Pressure	Noise Level dBas	Power Consumption wts.	Weight lbs	Height inches	Width inches	Depth inches
Briox PDQ	—	93	92	80	—	—	Flow Meter		43	265	44	17	15	16
Briox PDQ Plus		93		88		80	Flow Meter		43	300	54	25	15	16
Bunn R×O_2		93	85				Flow Meter	50	265	45	17½	13	10½	
Bunn 1000	95	95	95	93	85		Flow Meter		49	375	50	17½	14½	11½
Bunn 3001		90	85				Flow Meter	49	280	43	18½	13¾	13½	
Bunn Micro	93	90					Flow Meter	48	220	35	18½	12	13¾	
Creative Medical Ovation	93	93	90	80			Flow Meter		52	350	50	23	18	14½
Cryogenic Associates Roomate III	90±2	90±2	90±2	84±2			Rotary Restrictor	5.5	49	300	52	26	14	10
DeVilbiss DeVO/44	95	95	95	90	82		Flow Meter		49	390	44	23¾	15½	13
DeVilbiss DEVO/MC29	95	93	85				Flow Meter	8.5	49	265	29	21½	12½	14
DeVilbiss DeVO/MC29-90	95	95	90				Flow Meter	8.5	49	265	29	21½	12½	14
Erie Medical	95	95	95		85		Flow Meter		53	390	115	32	22	19
Erie Medical Eriette	94	94	90				Flow Meter	5.0	52	420	57	16	15	17
Health Pyne BX-3000	90±3	90±3	90±3	85±3			Flow Meter	5.0	52	340	55	17½	16½	22
Hospitak	92	92	85				Flow Meter		47	300	35	10	10½	16
Hudson 6400	93±3	93±3	93±3	90			Flow Meter	10.0	47	330	59	24¼	16¾	13½
Inspircon 3500	95±3	95±3	93±3	85±3			Flow Meter		49	351	45	15¾	12¼	17½
Inspircon 7500	95±3	95±3	93±3	85±3			Flow Meter		49	350	57	18½	14	19¾
Invacare Prime Air		95	92	90	85		Flow Meter	4.0	52	490	95	24	14½	20½
Invacare Prime Air-two		95			85		Flow Meter	4.0	52	490	95	25	14½	20½
Invacare Mobilaire II	95	95	92				Rotary Restrictor		52	390	59	18	23¼	14½
Invacare Modilair III	95±2	95±2	92±3				Rotary Restrictor	4.0	52	390	62	18	23¼	14½
Mada Medical RespO_2	96±3	95±3	90±3				Flow Meter		50	375	45	15¼	15½	17½
Mountain Medical Aspen	93±3	93±3					Flow Meter	5.0		200	42	21½	16½	12½
Mountain Medical Econo$_2$	95±3	95±3	95±3	95±3	90±3		Flow Meter	5.0	49	390	115	27	18	16
Mountain Medical MaxO_2	95±3	95±3	95±3	88±3			Flow Meter	5.0		325	49	23	14	11

Device						Control							
Mountain Medical MiniO$_2$	95	93	87			Flow Meter	5.	52	325	55	15¾	15	23
Mountain Medical Summit	95±3	95±3	95±3	93±3	85±3	Flow Meter	5.0		430	59	25	17	13
Mountain Medical Two$_2$	95±3	95±3	95±3	95±3	90±3	Flow Meter		49	390	118	32	18	16
OECO High-Humidity RT5	40					Flow Meter		45	225	110	30	14	16
OECO Junior	95	96				Flow Meter		47	200	58	30	14	14½
Penox BX-3000	90	90	85			Flow Meter		50	340	55	17½	16½	22
Penox MiniO$_2$	95	93				Flow Meter		52	325	55	15¾	15	23
Proto-Med GOC	95±2	95±3	90±3			Rotary Restrictor		50	390	60	30⅛	14	10
Puritan-Bennett Companion 492	95±3	95±3	95±3	92±3		Rotary Restrictor		50	330	47	24	12	16
Puritan-Bennett BioCareO$_2$	95	95	92			Flow Meter		50	330	47	24	12	16
Smith & Davis Oxycon SF2	94	92				Flow Meter		52	350	58	14⅛	14¾	21
Timetgr Criterion	90	93				Flow Meter		54	400	51	25¾	17½	14¼
TravoMed Travopak	94					Rotary Restrictor	5	39	220	30	16	21	6
Union Carbidee Maric 4	90					Rotary Restrictor		46	380	61.5	26	15	15

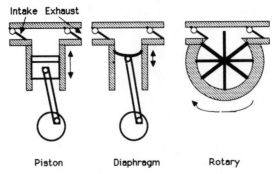

Figure 1.16 Types of air compressors.

high flows and/or high delivery pressures are required. As mentioned above, molecular-sieve oxygen concentrators often use a piston-type compressor to drive oxygen to the sieve beds and to supply an output pressure from the concentrator of 10–20 psig. Some piston compressors with air tank reservoirs have a pressure and flow capability sufficient to power mechanical ventilators and respirators.

The second type is the *diaphragm compressor* that works similarly to a piston compressor but has a flexible diaphragm in place of the piston. The motor moves the rod and diaphragm up and down. Air is drawn into the cylinder through the intake valve and exits through the exhaust valve, just as in the piston-type compressor. Diaphragm compressors are not capable of generating pressures or flows as high as those of the piston-type compressor, but diaphragm compressors are generally quieter and cause less vibration. The diaphragm-type compressor is used for powering medication nebulizers, larger volume pneumatic nebulizers, the Oxygen Enrichment, Ltd. concentrator, and the PortaBird IPPB device.

The third type of air compressor, the *rotary air compressor,* pumps air as a fan does. The vanes draw air in through the intake port and deliver the air out of the exhaust port. Small rotary compressors power the Bennett AP series of IPPB units, the Bennett MA-1 ventilator, and the Mountain Medical Econo$_2$ oxygen concentrator. Larger liquid-sealed devices can supply hospitals and other health care facilities with compressed air that is piped to the patient bedside. The liquid used to seal vanes is usually water, and *oil must not be used* in medical air compressors.

Table 1.3 lists specifications for some common air compressors used in respiratory home care.

A change in the noise level produced by an air compressor or the device's becoming hot to the touch is an indication that the compressor is in need of servicing. Output pressures and flow should be checked on a regular basis, and a preventive maintenance program outlined by the manufacturer or supplier should be followed.

Table 1.3. Specifications for Air Compressor

Compressors	Maximum Pressure	Maximum Flow	Power Requirement	Weight	H Outlets	Height	Width	Depth
1. Aridyne AD 2000	50 PSI	CF = 64L/M Reserve Flow 110L/M × 3 sec.	120 V 60 H$_2$ 12 amp	147 lbs (66.7 kg)	3	35″	17″	21″
2. Aridyne AD 3000	50 PSI	CF = 29L/M Reserve Flow 40L/M × 3 sec.	115 V 60 Hz 6 amp	73 lbs. (33 kg)	2	33.5″	11″	15⅛″
3. Aridyne AD 3500	50 PSI	42 LPM	120 V 60 Hz 8.5 amp.	90 lbs. (41 kg)	2	33.5″	11″	8″
4. Ohio High Performance	80 PSI	28L/M @ 50 PSI	120 V	49 lbs. (21.4 kg)	2	18″	9″	17″
5. Pulmo-Aide 561547 561648	20 PSI	12L/M	115 V 60 Hz 3 wire plug	6.5 lbs. (2.95 kg)	1	9″	5″	8″
6. Pulmo-Aide 561 series	20 PSI	12 L/M	115 V 60 Hz 1.5 amp	7.9 lbs (3.6 kg)	1	7.75″	9.75″	10″
7. Siemens	50 PSI	50 L/M	120 V 60 Hz 10 amp.	< 50 lbs (s̄ cart)	2	(s̄ cart) 15″ (c̄ cart) 19¼″	15¾″ 15¾″	11¾″ 11¾″
8. Timeter PSC-1	50 PSI	50L/M	120 V 60 c.y.A.C. 8 amp	approx. 33 lbs.	3	39″	18″	22″
9. Timeter PSC-4	50 PSI	7 L/M @ 50 PSI 20 L/M @ 20 PSI	115 V 60 Hz .8 HP	35 lbs. (15.9 kg)	1	12″	8″	19″
0. Timeter PSC-414	50 PSI	14 L/M @ 50 PSI 19 L/M @ 20 PSI	115 V 60 Hz .7 HP	30 lbs (13.6 kg)	1	11¾″	7¾″	18¾″
1. Timeter PSC-5	50 PSI	7 L/M @ 50 PSI 20 L/M @ 20 PSI	115 V 60 Hz .8 HP	15.5 lbs (7 kg)	1	10″	5″	9″

References

1. McPherson S. P. Respiratory therapy equipment. 3rd ed. St Louis: The CV Mosby Co., 1985.
2. Code of federal regulations: Title 49, Parts 1 to 199. Washington DC: US Government Printing Office, October 1973.
3. Compressed Gas Association. Handbook of compressed gases. New York: Reinhold, 1985.
4. Compressed Gas Association. Characteristics and handling of medical gases. 5th ed. New York: Compressed Gas Association, 1984.
5. National Fire Protection Association: Health care facilities, NFPA No. 99. New York: National Fire Protection Association, 1984.
6. National Fire Protection Association. Bulk oxygen systems. NFPA No. 50, New York: National Fire Protection Association, 1979.
7. Shigesko J. W, Bonekat H. W. The Current Status of Oxygen-Conserving Devices (editorial). Respiratory Care 1985; 30:833-836.
8. Union Carbide—Linde Division. Precautions and safe practices—Liquified atmospheric gases, New York: Union Carbide—Linde Division, 1979.
9. Union Carbide—Linde Division. Safe handling of liquid oxygen, nitrogen, and argon. New York: Union Carbide—Linde Division, 1980.
10. National Fire Protection Association. Nonflammable medical gas systems. NFPA No. 56F. New York: National Fire Protection Association, 1983.
11. Heinz P. D. The effect of high altitudes on oxygen concentrators. Rx Home Care 1985;7: 63–65, 89.

2 *Gas Pressure Regulators and Flow Controllers*

As discussed in the first chapter, a gas source is required for virtually all respiratory care setups. The gas source must be regulated, to ensure that the proper amount of gas is delivered to the patient. Three devices used to control the gas flow are the reducing valve, the flowmeter, and the pressure regulator. The pressure-reducing valve does only what its name implies—reduces pressure; the flowmeter controls flowrate; and a regulator both reduces pressure and controls flowrate. This chapter will discuss these three control mechanisms.

Reducing Valves

The most basic type of pressure-controlling device is a reducing valve. Initially, a reducing valve was used to lower a cylinder's high internal-gas pressure to a constant delivery pressure so that the cylinder gas could safely and accurately power other devices, usually at a pressure of 50 pounds per square inch gauge (psig). This is still the most common use for reducing valves, but they are now also used in liquid-oxygen systems, cylinder manifolds, compressed-air systems, and in other respiratory therapy devices, including pressure regulators.

Single-Stage Valve

Figure 2.1 shows the design of a simple, single-stage pressure reducing valve. Cylinder gas enters at the high-pressure inlet. The diaphragm in the center of the valve is kept upright by a balance of spring tension on the left and gas pressure on the right. If the gas pressure becomes lower than the spring tension against the diaphragm, the diaphragm and poppet valve are pushed to the right by the spring, opening the high-pressure inlet, and allowing gas to flow into the reducing valve from the cylinder. Once the gas pressure rises to equal the spring tension, the diaphragm returns to its upright position, and the poppet valve closes, stopping the flow of gas into the reducing valve from the cylinder. If the desired delivery pressure from the reducing valve is 50 psig, the spring tension against the diaphragm should be set at 50 psig so that the gas pressure will equilibrate on the other (delivery) side of the diaphragm at that pressure level. Some home care devices require a lower delivery pressure; for example, certain liquid systems require restrictors with a delivery pressure of 20 psig. It is crucial that the practitioner supply pressure-controlling devices with the proper delivery pressure or the safety and accuracy of devices they are to be attached to will be seriously compromised.

Multistage Valve

Another type of pressure-reducing valve is the multistage reducing valve that consists of two or more reducing valves (like the one described above) attached in series. The reducing valve described previously is referred to as a single-stage reducing valve because gas is reduced from cylinder pressure to delivery pressure in a single step. Multistage reducing valves reduce pressure to one pressure level in the first stage and to another pressure level in a second stage (Figure 2.2).

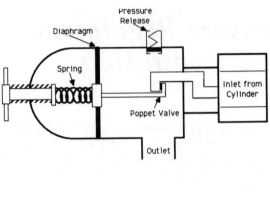

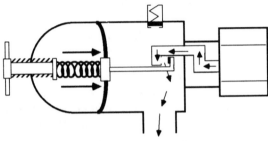

Figure 2.1 Single-stage pressure reducing valve. As gas pressure drops on the right side of the diaphragm, the spring tension pushes the diaphragm and poppet valve to the right, opening the gas inlet.

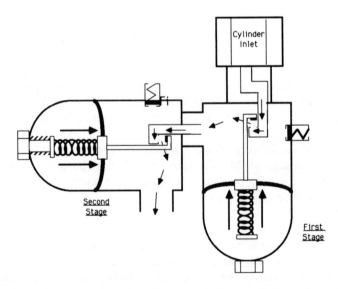

Figure 2.2 Multistage reducing valve. Composed of two reducing valves that reduce pressure in two stages.

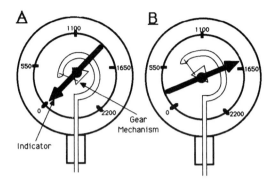 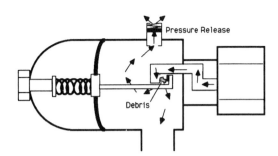

Figure 2.3 Bourdon-type pressure gauge. Under zero pressure the tube in the Bourdon gauge is coiled. As pressure is applied, the tube straightens, the gear mechanism rotates, and the needle indicates the pressure level on a calibrated scale.

Figure 2.4 Pressure release mechanism. A buildup of pressure beyond a set level within the reducing valve causes the release mechanism to vent, thereby protecting the patient and the equipment.

Multistage reducing valves are usually double- or triple-stage valves, their name referring to the number of steps (valves) by which they reduce pressure.

Gauge

On each reducing valve, cylinder pressure is displayed on a gauge, almost always a Bourdon-type gauge. The primary component of the Bourdon pressure gauge is a coiled tube (Figure 2.3). As a higher pressure is exerted on the inside of the tube, it tends to straighten; this response is due to the fact that the surface area of the upper side of the tube is greater than the surface area of the lower side. The second component of the gauge is a gear mechanism with an indicator needle attached. As the coil expands under higher pressure and straightens, the gear mechanism rotates the needle to indicate a higher contents pressure on the calibrated scale.

Pressure-Release Mechanism

A pressure-reducing valve has an internal pressure-release mechanism that is normally set for 50% higher than the delivery pressure (Figure 2.4). If a valve malfunction occurs, such as the poppet valve being kept open by debris, the pressure in the reducing valve will continue to rise above the delivery pressure as gas continues to enter from the cylinder. The pressure release will vent at its set level to protect the patient and equipment. If the malfunction corrects itself and the pressure falls to below the pressure-release setting, the pressure release will reseat.

NFPA Regulations

NFPA regulations that apply directly to reducing valves are as follows:[1]

- A pressure-reducing valve must be used on a high-pressure cylinder and must be listed for high-pressure service. It is hazardous to connect fixed or adjustable orifices, flowmeters, or other devices directly to a cylinder without a pressure-reducing valve or regulator.

- The reducing valve must conform to American Standard or Pin Index Safety System connections for cylinder valves, and the low-pressure outlet must conform to the Diameter Index Safety System or must be a low-pressure quick-connect valve of noninterchangeable design. Therefore, a reducing valve designed for use with one gas should not be used with another.

- Pressure-reducing valves must be labeled: **Oxygen—Use No Oil.** Connections on the cylinder valve and the reducing valve must be free of oil and grease, and the person making the connection must not have oil or grease on his hands, gloves, or clothing.

- A pressure-reducing valve is to be permanently labeled with the name of the gas for which it is intended, along with the name of the manufacturer or supplier.

- The following steps must be taken when connecting a reducing valve to a cylinder:

  1. Secure the cylinder by chain or strap to an immovable object, appropriate cart, or stand (see Chapter 1).
  2. Remove the protective cap.
  3. Verify cylinder contents by reading the label. The color code must match the contents label.
  4. Inspect the cylinder-valve outlet and the pressure-reducing valve to be sure they are not contaminated with foreign objects, oil, or grease.
  5. Turn the cylinder valve away from anyone present, stand to the side, and quickly open and close the valve to remove any dust that might be in the valve outlet. (This will create noise, and anyone present should be warned ahead of time.)
  6. Attach the pressure-reducing valve and tighten securely, using the appropriate wrench provided by the manufacturer or supplier. Do not use pipe wrenches, and do not force the reducing valve.
  7. Open the cylinder valve slowly to pressurize the reducing valve, then open it completely and turn it back one-fourth to one-half turn. The pressure-reducing valve should be closed when the cylinder is initially opened and whenever it is not in use.

- The pressure-reducing valve must be on a preventive maintenance program as recommended by the manufacturer. The reducing valve must be serviced by qualified personnel in a shop area designated for the servicing of oxygen equipment. The servicing area must be clean and free of oil and grease and not used for the repair of other equipment. Only service manuals, operators manuals, instructions, replacement parts, and procedures provided or recommended by the manufacturer are to be used.

- Reducing valves must not be sterilized with flammable sterilizing agents, such as ethylene oxide or alcohol. A significant hazard is associated with residual sterilizing agent left in the valve. Polyethylene must not be used to package a reducing valve for sterilization because polyethylene may slough particles that are pure hydrocarbons and thus constitute a serious fire hazard. Sterilizing agents must be oil free and must not damage components of the reducing valve. Cleaning a reducing valve by wiping it off with a cloth and mild soap or disinfectant that is not damaging to plastics is usually sufficient.

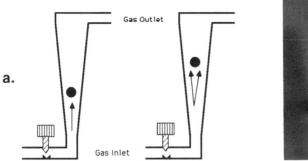
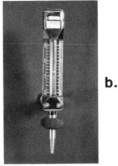

Figure 2.5 A Thorpe Tube Flowmeter. The ball float is pushed upwards by incoming gas molecules. Flowrate is indicated by the position of the ball against a corresponding calibrated scale. **B** Picture of Puritan-Bennett Flowmeter (Thorpe-type). Our grateful thanks to Puritan-Bennett's Portable Ventilator Division, Boulder, Colorado, for their assistance in helping us develop material.

Flowmeters

After the cylinder-gas pressure is reduced to the appropriate level, the control of the gas flow-rate is frequently required. Flow-metering devices or flowmeters are used.

Thorpe Tube

The most common type is the Thorpe tube flowmeter, which is composed of a needle valve, a ball float, and a tube that gradually increases in diameter from bottom to top (Figures 2.5A and 2.5B). Flow is controlled by the gradual opening and closing of the needle valve, and the Thorpe tube and float measure the flow. As more gas passes the needle valve, the force of the gas molecules hitting the bottom of the float increases, pushing the ball float upwards to a point where the diameter of the tube is large enough to allow the gas molecules to flow around the ball.

A Thorpe tube flowmeter can be one of two designs (Figure 2.6). A tube that does not compensate for back pressure (uncompensated) has the needle valve upstream, ahead of the tube and float, with the tube calibrated at atmospheric pressure. If a restriction is placed downstream from the float, causing back pressure, the molecules in the gas are compressed closer together; thus more molecules get past the float than normally would without the back pressure and the density of the gas is increased. Then as the molecules pass the restriction, they expand to atmospheric pressure, forming a larger amount of gas than that measured by the flowmeter. *So the reading is lower than actual flow.* The resistance offered by the jets found in medication nebulizers, large volume nebulizers, and entrainment devices will cause this inaccuracy.

A Thorpe tube flowmeter that compensates for back pressure (compensated) has the needle valve downstream, past the tube and float, so the tube is calibrated at delivery pressure (usually 50 psig). This type of flowmeter remains accurate when a restriction is placed downstream, because the tube and float are already exposed to maximum delivery pressure and further compression of the gas and increased gas density cannot occur.

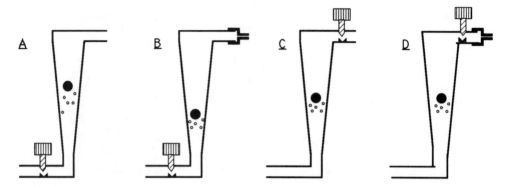

Figure 2.6 Uncompensated and compensated Thorpe Tube Flowmeters. The needle valve is located upstream from the tube and ball float in a non-back-pressure-compensated tube (A & B) and downstream from the tube and float in a back-pressure-compensated tube (C & D). In an uncompensated tube with a restriction downstream from the tube and float (B), back pressure will lessen the lift effect on the float (because the tube is calibrated at atmospheric pressure) and the flow reading will be rendered inaccurate. In a back-pressure-compensated flowmeter, a restriction downstream from the float (D) does not affect the flow reading, as the tube is already calibrated at gas delivery pressure.

The key to whether a flowmeter is back-pressure compensated is the location of the needle valve—it's upstream from the tube in a non-back-pressure-compensated flowmeter and downstream from the tube in a back-pressure-compensated flowmeter. However, because the location of the valve can be difficult to determine by looking at the exterior of the flowmeter and because even an apparent location can be deceiving, two other ways of determining flowmeter design can be used. The first way is to look at the label. On a back-pressure-compensated flowmeter, the label will indicate that the flowmeter was calibrated at 50 pounds per square inch gauge (psig) pressure and will also state the temperature at which the calibration was performed; whereas on a non-back-pressure-compensated flowmeter, the label will indicate that the flowmeter was calibrated at atmospheric pressure. The second way to determine whether a flowmeter is back-pressure compensated is to see what happens to the float when the flowmeter is connected to a pressurized source. This should be done in the following manner: With the flowmeter turned off, connect it to the reducing valve, and turn the cylinder on to effect pressurization. Because a back-pressure-compensated flowmeter has the needle valve downstream from the tube, the float will rise as the tube is pressurized and then will return to the bottom. In the non-back-pressure-compensated flowmeter, the float will not move because the tube is at atmospheric pressure, with the closed needle valve between the pressurized gas source and the float.

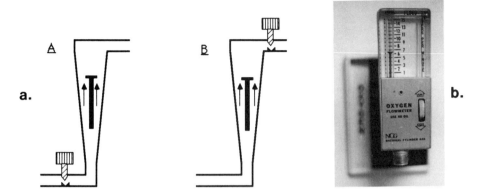

Figure 2.7 A Kinetic flowmeters. A, non-back-pressure-compensated. B, Back-pressure-compensated. A plunger replaces the ball float of the Thorpe tube flowmeter. **B** Picture of NCG Flowmeter (Kinetic-type).

Kinetic

Another type of flowmeter, similar in design to the Thorpe tube, is the kinetic flowmeter. This device has a plunger instead of a ball float and can also be either back-pressure compensated or non-back-pressure compensated (Figures 2.7A and 2.7B), depending upon the location of the needle valve. The same methods as those listed for the Thorpe tube device may be used in determining whether the kinetic flowmeter is back-pressure compensated or not.

Recently, some manufacturers have introduced flowmeters that are capable of delivering small flows (e.g. 1/4, 1/2 or 0.1, 0.2 L/min). The supplier should be cautioned that tests run in our laboratories indicate that not all brands of flowmeters are capable of accurately measuring these low flows. All flowmeters, especially the newer low-flow versions, should be tested against a calibrated Thorpe tube laboratory rotometer or similar device—first, before being placed into service and then periodically thereafter as part of a preventive maintenance program, with records of test results being maintained.

NFPA Standards

The NFPA standards that relate directly to flowmeters and other flow-metering devices are as follows:[1]

1. A flowmeter must not be connected directly to a cylinder without a pressure-reducing valve in place.
2. Because calibration and function are dependent upon gas density, the flowmeter label must show the proper supply pressure. Figure 2.8 demonstrates the inaccuracy that occurs when a flowmeter is operated at a delivery pressure other than the one for which it was designed.

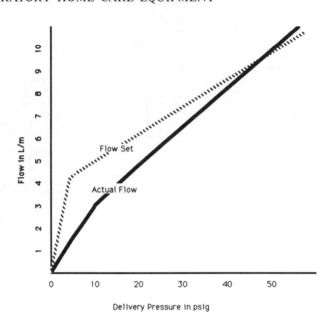

Figure 2.8 Relative accuracy of flowmeters and flow restrictors at varying delivery pressures for devices designed for use at 50 psig.

3. Flowmeters must be labeled with the warning: **"Oxygen—Use No Oil"** and with the name of the manufacturer or supplier.
4. Flowmeters must be serviced in the same manner described for reducing valves. They must be serviced by qualified personnel in a shop area designated for the servicing of oxygen equipment. The servicing area must be clean and free of oil and grease and not used for the repair of other equipment. Only service manuals, operators manuals, instructions, replacement parts, and procedures provided or recommended by the manufacturer are to be used.
5. Because a flowmeter operates at a pressure lower than 60 psig, it may be sterilized with nonflammable mixtures containing ethylene oxide and carbon dioxide or fluorocarbon diluents if necessary. However, polyethylene must not be used in the packaging of a flowmeter, and the sterilizing agent must be oil free and must not damage the materials that make up the flowmeter. Wiping a flowmeter off with a cloth and mild soap or disinfectant that is not damaging to plastics is sufficient in most circumstances.

Regulators

As mentioned at the beginning of this chapter, a regulator controls pressure and measures flow. One type of regulator is a combination reducing valve and Thorpe tube or kinetic flowmeter. The reducing valve controls the pressure, usually to 50 psig, and the flowmeter is used for achieving the desired flow.

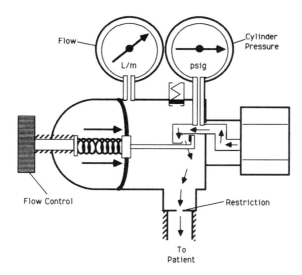

Figure 2.9 Bourdon Regulator. Bourdon regulator, consisting of a set-sized orifice and an adjustable pressure-reducing valve. One of the Bourdon gauges monitor cylinder-gas pressure; the other gauge monitors valve upstream from the restriction and displays the corresponding flowrate in liters per minute. The Bourdon regulator is not back-pressure compensated, so any downstream restriction will render the flow inaccurate.

A second type of regulator is a Bourdon-type device (Figure 2.9). A Bourdon regulator consists of a set-sized orifice and an adjustable pressure-reducing valve. The pressure-reducing valve alters the pressure delivered to the fixed restriction (set-sized orifice) and therefore adjusts the pressure gradient and the resulting flow across the restriction. Flow is directly related to the pressure gradient across a fixed orifice; therefore, if the pressure downstream from the restriction always remains atmospheric, the pressure upstream, above the restriction, relates directly to the flowrate across it. The Bourdon regulator employs two Bourdon gauges: One monitors cylinder gas pressure; the other monitors pressure upstream from the restriction and displays, in liters per minute (lpm), the flowrate that relates to the pressure and therefore to the pressure gradient that will result across the orifice to atmospheric pressure.

The Bourdon regulator is not back-pressure compensated. Any downstream resistance that causes back pressure will render the reading inaccurate. When resistance is added to a Bourdon regulator, the pressure downstream from the restriction is no longer atmospheric and the pressure gradient and flow across the restriction drops, resulting in an actual flow that is less than the flow reading (Figure 2.10). Figure 2.11 shows the relative accuracy of the compensated and uncompensated devices that have been described.

Jet nebulizers and other small restrictions and extra-long connecting tubing must be avoided when using a Bourdon regulator, especially at low flows. The pressure against the Bourdon regulator orifice is low at low-settings, and long tubing can cause enough resistance to make the flow

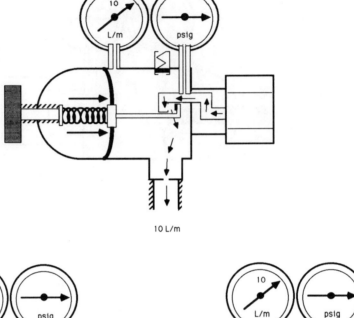

10 L/m

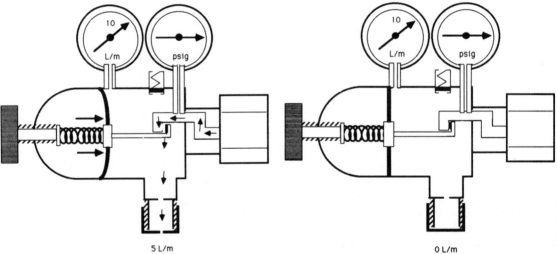

5 L/m   0 L/m

Figure 2.10 Resistance added to a Bourdon-type regulator.

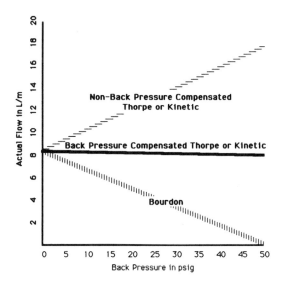

Figure 2.11 Accuracy of types of flowmeters.

reading inaccurate. If in doubt, one should use a Thorpe tube flow tester, such as the one produced by Erie Medical, to measure the flow at the patient end of the connecting tubing to be sure the flow the patient is receiving corresponds to the Bourdon-gauge setting.

The selection of a regulator depends on the manner in which the device will be used. The Bourdon-gauge reading will remain accurate in any position, such as lying on its side, as long as no back pressure is applied to it. If restrictions are likely to be placed downstream from the Bourdon regulator, it is a poor choice. In fact, nonkinkable connecting tubing should be standard because the Bourdon regulator will display the set flowrate even if the connecting tubing is totally occluded and no flow is going to the patient. The uncompensated flowmeter should be avoided because in the presence of back pressure it can deliver higher flows than indicated. This is especially important in treating patients with chronic obstructive pulmonary disease (COPD), as they may hypoventilate and retain more CO_2 if the flow of oxygen is elevated. Compensated Thorpe tube and kinetic flowmeters are accurate, once set, in all positions. However, the reading will not be accurate if the flowmeter is moved from its normal vertical position. If the device is laid on its side and the needle valve is accidentally turned, the flowrate will change, and determining this visually will be impossible without returning the flowmeter to its upright position.

For this discussion of gas regulators and controllers to be complete, the needle-valve type of gas regulator (Figure 2.12) must be mentioned. This device may still be found in home care and adjusts flow directly from the cylinder, with no reducing valve in place. Because cylinder pressure drops continuously as the gas is removed, the actual flow past the needle valve drops also. The

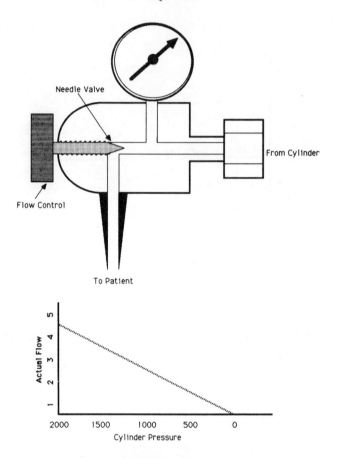

Figure 2.12 Needle valve type regulator.

drop in flow is proportional to the decrease in cylinder pressure and the corresponding decline in the pressure gradient across the needle valve. Thus, this type of regulator is not accurate and has no place in quality home care.

Because a regulator is composed of both a reducing valve and a flowmeter, the standards described above for both devices apply to all regulators.

Flow Restrictors

The flow restrictor (Figures 2.13A, 2.13B, 2.13C and 2.13D) is now available as an alternative to the flowmeter in the home care setting. One type of restrictor is the fixed orifice, which provides a set flow; if the flow must be changed, a restrictor of another size is required. Another type is the adjustable restrictor, which rotates to provide several orifices and flowrates. Because the adjustable restrictor provides set-sized restrictions that can be calibrated, as opposed to the variable-sized restriction allowed by a needle valve, a tube and float for measuring flow are eliminated.

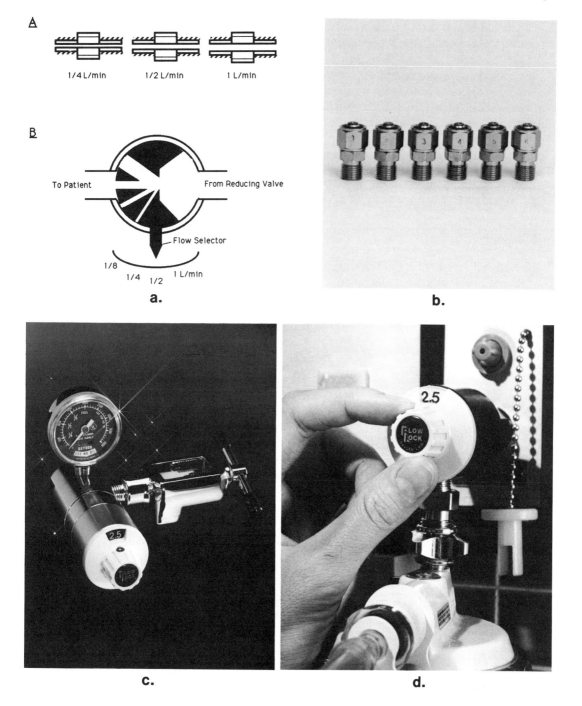

Figure 2.13 A Flow restrictors. A. Set-sized restrictors. B. Adjustable restrictor. **B** Flow restrictors. Courtesy of Erie Medical. **C** Flowlook adjustable restrictor and regulator. Courtesy of Lifeguard Medical Products. **D** Wall mount flow lock adjustable restrictors. Courtesy of Lifeguard Medical Products.

It should be noted that tests in our laboratories indicate that not all brands of restrictors are accurate. Therefore, the supplier should check all such devices with a calibrated Thorpe tube or similar measuring device before they are placed into service, should recheck them periodically, and should keep proper records.

Some restrictors are designed for use at 50 psig pressure, whereas others are designed to operate at a pressure of 20 psig, such as those in liquid-oxygen devices; thus, according to NFPA standards, restrictors must be marked with the service pressure for which they were designed. Figure 2.8 demonstrates the inaccuracy that occurs when a flow restrictor is operated at a delivery pressure other than that for which it was designed.

Flow restrictors fall into the category of flowmeters and must meet the same standards. A flow restrictor combined with a reducing valve offers a new variety of regulator; both devices must meet the NFPA requirements listed in this chapter.

References

1. National Fire Protection Association. Health Care Facilities, NFPA No. 99. New York: National Fire Protection Association, 1984.

3 Gas Administration and Monitoring Devices

Gas administration in the home can frequently be accomplished by using simple devices such as oxygen cannulas, catheters, masks, or enclosures. At times, other more complex devices, such as air entrainment devices or oxygen percentage controllers, are necessary to control the percentage of oxygen dispensed precisely. Also, monitoring devices are frequently used to check or monitor oxygen delivery or breathing patterns. This chapter will discuss all of these types of devices.

Oxygen Masks

Simple Mask

The original style of oxygen mask developed by Ingenhouse in 1789 is still widely used today and is called a simple mask.[1] The simple mask is designed to receive oxygen into a modified cone-shaped face piece that covers the patient's nose and mouth (Figure 3.1). As the patient inhales, the oxygen in the mask and the incoming oxygen flow is breathed in along with air drawn through the exhalation ports. Some brands include an air-dilution port on the oxygen inlet to draw in some room air as oxygen enters the mask (Figure 3.2). In theory, the increased flow into the mask reduces the carbon dioxide build-up in the mask during the exhalation period.

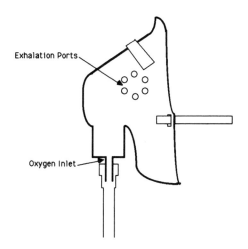

Figure 3.1 Simple oxygen mask.

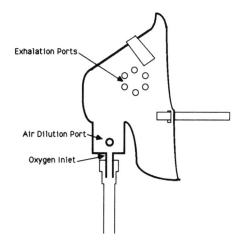

Figure 3.2 Simple oxygen mask with air dilution port.

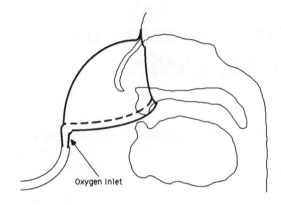

Oxygen Inlet

Figure 3.3 Face shield.

A simple mask can be connected directly to the flowmeter or regulator by way of a connecting tubing and an oxygen connector, which is sometimes referred to as a "Christmas tree" due to its configuration and green color. Humidifiers are also used in the treatment of some patients for comfort because it's easier to breathe moist air. Generally, it is preferable to use a simple mask with an oxygen connector, especially at relatively low flows, unless the patient complains of dryness and then a humidifier can be added. Humidifiers that are used should be checked for gas leaks and must have an audible pressure relief (see Chapter 4).

The oxygen percentage delivered by a simple mask generally ranges from 35–55%, but can vary significantly with changes in the patient's ventilatory pattern and the resulting changes in peak inspiratory flow and minute volume. These changes can occur during exercise or as a result of apprehension or the worsening of their disease process. Prior to use, a minimum flow of oxygen into the simple mask is necessary to flush previously exhaled carbon dioxide.

Face Shield

One variation of the simple mask is the face shield, which rests on the bridge of the nose and then angles out away from the chin (Figure 3.3). This design provides a large opening between the mask and the patient's chin so that speaking and drinking are possible without removing the mask. Oxygen enters the mask through a series of delivery ports in the lower portion of the mask, and room air is drawn in through the large opening. Oxygen percentages are similar to those for the traditional style of simple mask.

The face tent rests on the patient's chin and is open at the top, away from the face.

Nasal Mask

Another variation of the simple mask is the nasal mask. The nasal mask (Figure 3.4) is constructed as a smaller version of the typical simple mask and only covers the nose. Just as in the simple mask, oxygen enters the mask and the patient inhales the oxygen within the mask, the incoming flow of oxygen, and room air through the exhalation ports. An advantage of using the nasal mask is that the patient is able to speak or drink without removing the mask.

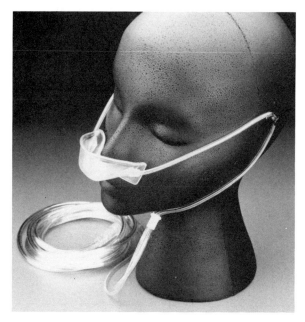

Figure 3.4 Nasal mask. Courtesy of Marquest Medical Products, Inc. Englewood, Colorado.

Partial Rebreathing Mask

When oxygen percentages are needed that are slightly higher than the range for a simple mask, a partial rebreathing mask can be used. The first partial rebreathing mask (the BLB mask) was introduced in 1938 at the Mayo Clinic by Boothby, Lovelace, and Bulbulian.[2] The partial rebreathing mask in use today employs a face mask that is essentially the same as the simple mask with the addition of a reservoir bag (Figure 3.5). The incoming source gas is directed into the reservoir bag and when the patient inhales, he theoretically first draws gas from the mask and bag, and then through the exhalation ports. During exhalation, he exhales approximately the first one-third (which is high in oxygen and low in carbon dioxide because it was the portion of gas in the upper airways and not directly exposed to gas exchange) into the reservoir bag. The remainder of exhaled gases exits through the exhalation ports. The partial rebreathing mask should have sufficient flow into it to prevent the reservoir bag from completely collapsing during inspiration. Oxygen concentrations up to 60% can be obtained with a disposable partial rebreathing mask and up to 75% with the permanent BLB type.[3]

Nonrebreathing Mask

The nonrebreathing mask is used when very high oxygen percentages or special mixtures with controlled oxygen percentages are required. The design of the nonrebreathing mask (Figure 3.6) employs a reservoir like the partial rebreathing mask plus the addition of one-way valves on the

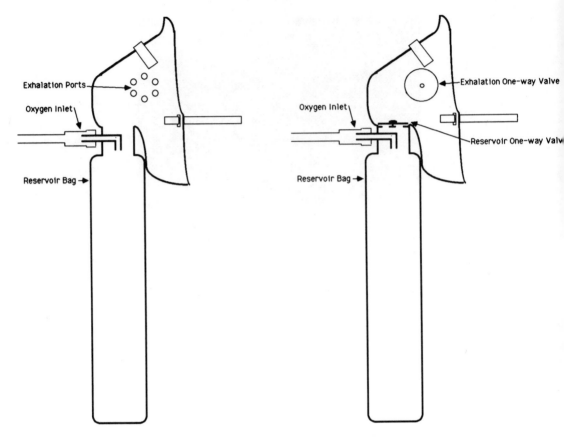

Figure 3.5 Partial rebreathing mask.   **Figure 3.6** Nonrebreathing mask.

exhalation ports and between the reservoir bag and the mask. These one-way valves allow oxygen to enter only from the reservoir bag and permit the exhaled gas to exit only out the exhalation ports. Permanent, tight-fitting, nonrebreathing masks can deliver virtually 100% of the source gas being delivered. Disposable masks can be expected to deliver 60–70% oxygen or source gas, because the fit is not as snug as nondisposables and some masks lack valves that cover both sets of exhalation ports. The missing valve is one method of allowing a safety inlet port in the event of oxygen delivery system failure. When approximately 100% oxygen or other source gas is required, a tight, well-fitting mask is necessary where both sets of exhalation ports are covered with valves, and the safety gas inlet is a spring/disc type. If a disposable mask with this design, which seals well, is not available, a permanent unit is preferred to maximize the oxygen percentage. As described with the partial rebreathing mask, the flow of gas being delivered should be adjusted so that the reservoir bag does not collapse completely during inspiration.

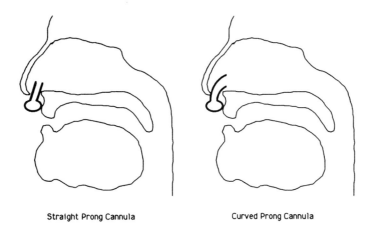

Straight Prong Cannula   Curved Prong Cannula

Figure 3.7 Nasal oxygen cannulas. (Straight prong and curved prong.)

Oxygen Cannula

The oxygen cannula consists of two prongs that direct oxygen into the two nares (Figure 3.7). There are two primary types of designs for nasal oxygen cannulas. The first type utilizes two straight tubes, while in the other type the prongs curve posteriorly and increase in diameter. It is felt that the curved-prong type may be useful for higher flows as the oxygen is directed more posteriorly toward the turbinates as opposed to upward toward the opening of the frontal sinuses as with the straight prong-type. The curved, increasing diameter style is also considered quieter in operation. Oxygen cannulas are now available from Salter Labs in a clear model for inconspicuous use with the home care patient, as well as in pediatric and neonatal sizes.

Two cannulas recently introduced by ESP are the oxy-frame (Figure 3.8A) and the head/ nocturnal cannula (Figure 3.8B), both designed for comfort and practicality.

With oxygen flows as high as 8 L/min, oxygen percentages of up to 50% can be achieved with an oxygen cannula, but the actual percentages may vary markedly from patient to patient.[2] Flows approaching 8 L/min can irritate, especially with the straight-prong-style cannula. Flows of 1/8 to 4 L/min have been successfully used to provide controlled oxygen delivery.[2] As described earlier, it is especially important to test low-flow flowmeters for accuracy in long-term, low flow oxygen delivery.

The use of low-flow oxygen in the home has raised the question of whether there's a need to use humidifiers with oxygen cannulas. Due to the inherent problems associated with humidifiers (gas leaks, contamination, spilling water, unreliable audible pressure-releases, etc.), it is better to provide low flow oxygen without humidification unless comfort becomes a significant issue. Bypassing the humidification devices has had another liability until recently. An occluded oxygen-connecting tubing could go unnoticed without the audible pressure release found on most humidifiers. The use of non-kinkable connecting oxygen tubing has greatly reduced this problem, and

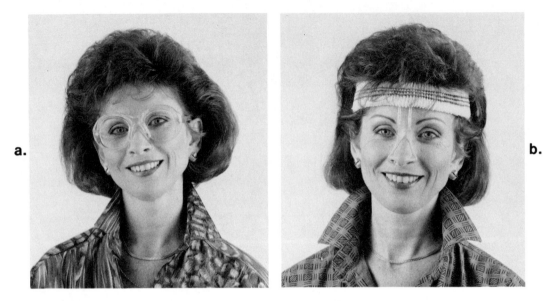

Figure 3.8 A Oxyframe cannula. Courtesy of ESP. **B** Head / nocturnal cannula. Courtesy of ESP.

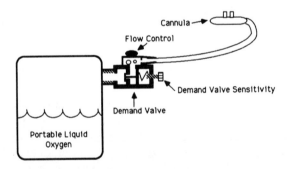

Figure 3.9 Pulse oxygen delivery system.

more recently an audible pressure-release with a rotor to provide a visual indication of flow, called the FlowAlert, has been introduced by Precision Medical. The FlowAlert attaches between the flowmeter or reducing valve and the oxygen connecting tubing and is functional for flows above 1 L/min.

Nasal oxygen cannulas are also employed in conjunction with the pulse- flow liquid oxygen unit Demand Oxygen Controller, DOC® (Figure 3.9) which is manufactured by CRYO$_2$, where the liquid unit acts as a demand valve and delivers oxygen in response to the patient's inspiratory effort. Other pulse/demand-oxygen units are available that can be used with cylinders, concentrators, or liquid systems. The Demand Oxygen Saver System (DO$_2$S®) and the Chad Therapeutics Oxymatic® are designed to work with portable systems.

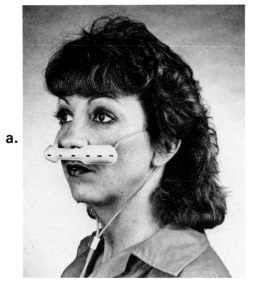

a.

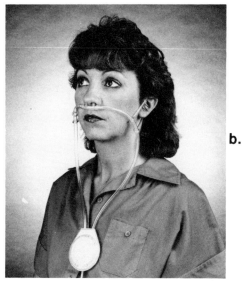

b.

Figure 3.10 A Oxymizer cannula. Courtesy of Chad Therapeutics. **B** Oxymizer Pendant cannula. Courtesy of Chad Therapeutics.

Another new approach to the conservation of oxygen when using a nasal cannula are the two versions of the Oxymizer® (Figures 3.10A and 3.10B). The first type of Oxymizer® has a small diaphragm within the base of the cannula itself. During exhalation, oxygen flows into the base of the cannula and displaces the diaphragm and collects oxygen. Then during inhalation, the patient draws oxygen from the reservoir in the base of the cannula as well as the incoming oxygen flow and room air. The second design of this unit is configured as a pendant which acts as the reservoir. Oxygen inters the pendant and displaces a diaphragm again providing a reservoir for oxygen to be inhaled during the next breath.

Cleaning and Disinfection—Oxygen cannulas should be cleaned with mild soap that does not leave a soap film and disinfected every week or two as needed with a disinfectant that is suitable for oxygen administration devices to keep the cannula clean and free of debris. Cannulas should be replaced every two to four weeks, or more frequently if necessary. If a humidifier is used, it should be cleaned and disinfected at least weekly in the same manner as the oxygen cannula.

Safety—All safety requirements for oxygen administration sites must be observed when administering oxygen by mask or cannula (see Chapter 1).

Oxygen Catheters

The first nasal oxygen catheter was introduced by Sir Arbuthnot Lane in 1907.[3] The oxygen catheter consists of a tube that has a series of openings in the distal end. It must be color coded green to help in differentiating it from a feeding tube.[5] The catheter is inserted through the nose into the pharynx and the tip should be positioned just behind the uvula (Figures 3.11A and 3.11B).

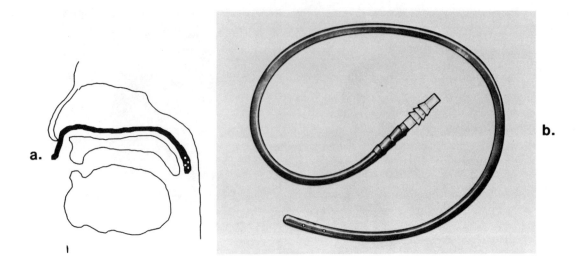

Figure 3.11 A Nasal catheter. **B** Oxygen catheter. Courtesy of Hudson Oxygen Therapy Sales Company, Temecula, CA.

Nasal catheters use the pharynx as an internal oxygen reservoir, but studies have failed to show significant differences in blood gas levels in patients receiving comparable flows of oxygen with an oxygen cannula.[6,7]

Prior to insertion, the catheter should be lubricated with a just enough petroleum jelly to lightly coat the surface of the catheter. Water soluble jelly has also been used but the catheter is more easily removed when petroleum jelly is used as the lubricant. Set the flowrate of oxygen to be delivered and inspect the exit ports at the distal end of the catheter to assure their patency. The distance from the ear lobe to the tip of the patient's ear will provide a guide as to the insertion depth. The catheter is gently inserted posteriorly along the floor of the nose. The catheter should never be forced. If obstruction is met, withdraw the catheter and attempt insertion in the other side of the nose. As the catheter is inserted, directly visualize the oral pharynx and once the catheter is visible past the uvula, stop inserting and draw the catheter back until it is again hidden. The catheter is then taped across the bridge of the nose. When direct visualization is not possible, the oxygen flowrate can be moderately elevated and the catheter may be inserted until the patient starts to gulp air. The catheter is then retracted approximately one inch. A new oxygen catheter should be placed into the opposite nare every 8 hours and the old one disposed of. Oxygen catheters should be used with caution in patients with ineffective epiglottic reflexes or epiglottal paralysis because the oxygen may be directed down the esophagus and result in serious gastric distention. If gastric distention occurs, the nasal catheter should be removed and another administration device employed. Since dry oxygen is delivered directly into the pharynx, a humidifier should be used with an oxygen catheter.

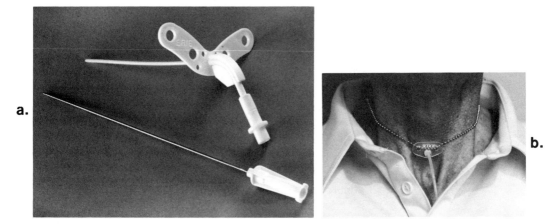

Figure 3.12 A Trachetter transtacheal oxygen catheter. Courtesy of the Institute for Transtracheal Oxygen Therapy, Presbyterian Denver Hospital, Denver CO. **B** Scoop Transtracheal oxygen catheter. Courtesy of the Institute for Transtracheal Oxygen Therapy, Presbyterian Denver Hospital, Denver CO.

Transtracheal Devices

A new application of catheters for oxygen administration utilizes a transtracheal oxygen catheter. The Trachette® or SCOOP® catheter (Figures 3.12A and 3.12B) is inserted through the tracheal wall, and oxygen is administered directly into the trachea. This technique has been shown to reduce flowrate requirement and provides a method of oxygen administration that is less conspicuous and eliminates the nasopharyngeal irritation that may result from nasal cannulas in some patients. Accidental removal of the device should be guarded against, and an alternate method of oxygen delivery should be accessible in the event of inadvertent removal of the transtracheal catheter.

Safety—All safety requirements outlined in Chapter 1 for oxygen administration sites apply to the administration of oxygen when using a catheter.

Oxygen Enclosures

Oxygen Tent

The original type of oxygen enclosure was the oxygen tent. The first oxygen tent was designed by Leonard Hill in 1920. However, the oxygen tent as we know it today, along with the ability to control the environment within the tent, is credited to Alvin Barach who added ice and a fan for cooling in 1924.[1] With the development of other oxygen-delivery devices, oxygen tents find little application in respiratory home care today and are generally reserved as a last choice due to their size, difficulty in cleaning, and the general complexity compared to other methods. However, oxygen tents offer improved stability of oxygen percentage, improved temperature control, better control of the aerosol content, and improved filtration of the environmental gases.

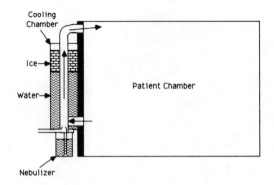

Figure 3.13 Croup oxygen tent.

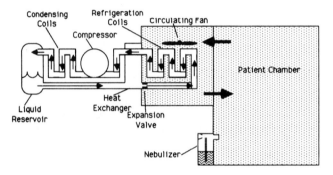

Figure 3.14 Refrigeration-type oxygen tent.

Ice as a Cooling Mechanism—There are basically two types of oxygen tents. One type uses ice as a cooling mechanism to remove body heat from the environment within the tent canopy, much as Alvin Barach's original tent did. These croup tents, such as the Croupette® units produced by Air Shields® utilize ice for cooling as do the disposable croup tents from Peace® Medical. Ice is used to cool the head partition of the croup tent and the tubing pathway through which aerosol enters (Figure 3.13). These enclosures have a relatively small internal volume and ice is sufficient to remove the heat from the circulating environment. Because of the relatively small volume within the canopy, flows from 8–12 L/min are sufficient to eliminate carbon dioxide build up and to maintain a relatively stable oxygen concentration. A pneumatic jet nebulizer is generally employed in the croup style tents to deliver both oxygen and aerosol.

Refrigeration Units—The second type of oxygen tent utilizes a refrigeration unit to remove the heat from the tent environment. Gas from within the canopy is circulated past refrigeration coils (Figure 3.14) either by means of entrainment or by the use of a fan. Refrigeration coils are used for larger volume canopies where ice is not sufficient to cool the environment adequately. Since the refrigeration coils are exposed to aerosol from within the canopy environment, the coils must be disinfected along with the nebulizer and tubing. One variation of the use of refrigeration coils

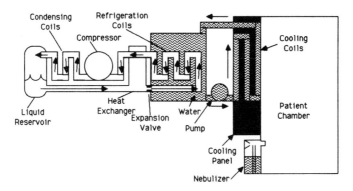

Figure 3.15 CAM oxygen tent.

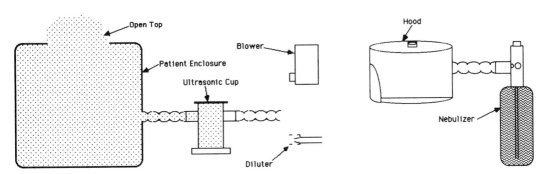

Figure 3.16 Open top tent.   **Figure 3.17** Oxygen hood.

is in the CAM® tent produced by Mistogen (Timeter). The refrigeration system is used to cool distilled water (Figure 3.15) which is then circulated through the head panel of the unit. Since the refrigeration coils do not come into contact with the patient environment, only the head panel needs to be cleaned and disinfected along with the nebulizer between patients. Due to the larger canopy volumes of these types of oxygen tents, higher flows (up to 15 L/min or higher) are required to maintain a stable oxygen level and to minimize the carbon dioxide level within the canopy.

Open Top Tents—In an effort to eliminate the need for refrigeration systems, the open top tent was designed (Figure 3.16). Heat rises out of the top of the tent canopy and higher flows (20–40 L/min) are used to keep the heat within the canopy from increasing.

Oxygen Hoods—The oxygen hood for infants was patterned after the open top tent, but encloses only the patient's head facilitating care of the infant, and was called an oxygen halo. Hoods have a closed or removable top and are constructed of clear plastic that must be noncombustible.[5] Due to the small internal gas volume, the flow from the nebulizer is sufficient to remove heat.

Pneumatic nebulizers are generally used to supply the desired oxygen percentage to the hood (Figure 3.17) along with aerosol. For oxygen percentages below the range of pneumatic nebulizers, two methods can be used (Figure 3.18).

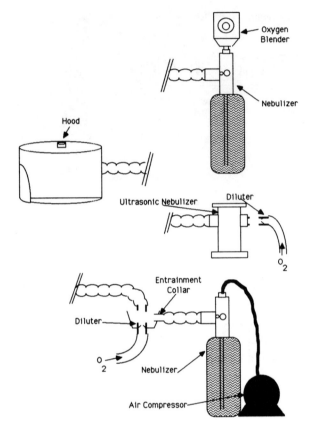

Figure 3.18 Oxygen delivery options for a hood.

One way is to set the nebulizer on the 100% setting and supply the required oxygen percentage from an air/oxygen controller (blender). In the home, this method requires additional amounts of equipment, such as oxygen and air cylinders or high output compressors.

Another way is with an entrainment device which delivers the required oxygen percentage to the hood, while the nebulizer is powered by a small air compressor and the aerosol is entrained by the entrainment device delivering aerosol into the hood along with the set oxygen percentage. This method, however, creates high noise levels. Another option is to use an ultrasonic nebulizer to supply aerosol to be carried into the enclosure by the entrainment device.

In general, flows of 5–15 L/min have been reported to be sufficient for oxygen hoods, although larger enclosures could require higher flows.[2,8] The noise level in hoods has also been reported as a problem and special care should be taken, such as using oxygen blenders to drive nebulizers so that they can be set on the 100% setting and the entrainment noise eliminated.[9-11] Cooling of the

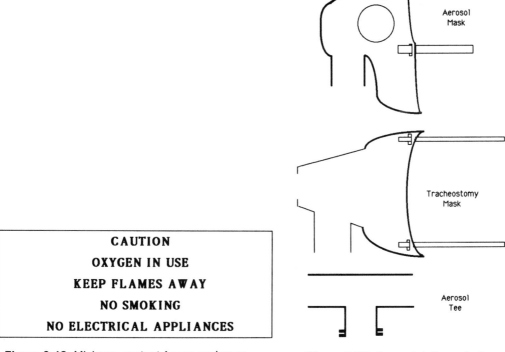

Figure 3.20 Aerosol delivery devices.

```
CAUTION

OXYGEN IN USE

KEEP FLAMES AWAY

NO SMOKING

NO ELECTRICAL APPLIANCES
```

Figure 3.19 Minimum content for an enclosure label.

infant has been reported to increase oxygen consumption so temperature monitoring may be required in small infants;[12] however, heated aerosol or heated humidity should not be added to the hood. If temperature control is required, it should be accomplished by providing a warmed total environment such as with an incubator or infant warmer. Hoods should be cleaned with a mild, non-film producing soap and then disinfected with a disinfectant suitable for the hood material.

Safety Requirements—All of the previously discussed safety requirements apply to the use of oxygen enclosures, including those for oxygen administration sites, and specifically those for enclosures (see Chapter 1). All enclosures must have a label on the interior visible to the patient and two or more labels on opposing sides of the exterior of the enclosure that are visible to occupants of the room.[5] Figure 3.19 shows the minimum context for an oxygen enclosure label.

Other Aerosol Delivery Devices

Other administration devices are utilized in the administration of aerosol besides enclosures. One is an aerosol mask that resembles a simple oxygen mask with larger inlet and outlet ports (Figure 3.20). Due to the reduced resistance of the aerosol masks inlet and outlet ports, this type of mask is frequently used with entrainment devices for controlled oxygen percentage delivery.

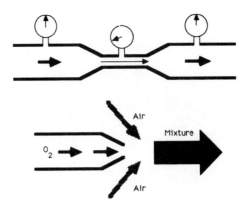

Figure 3.21 Bernoulli's principle.

Another device is a tracheostomy mask resembling a small dome which can be placed over the tracheostomy to deliver aerosols (Figure 3.20). Both aerosol and tracheostomy masks come in adult and pediatric sizes. A third device is an aerosol tee that can provide a direct connection to endotracheal tubes and some types of tracheostomy tubes (Figure 3.20). A more complete description of the use of these devices is found in Chapter 4.

Entrainment Devices

Entrainment devices utilize the Bernoulli's principle by using a jet (Figure 3.21) that lowers the lateral pressure of the oxygen source gas below atmospheric pressure so that air is entrained. The delivered oxygen percentage can be controlled by altering the size of the jet orifice or by changing the entrainment port size. It should be noted that these devices are often called Venturi masks, but the name is not correct since they do not contain a Venturi tube.

Most entrainment devices (diluters) alter the jet size to control oxygen percentage (Figures 3.22A, 3.22B and 3.22C). The smaller the jet size, the lower the lateral pressure that is created, hence, the more air that is entrained and the lower the oxygen percentage of the air/oxygen mixture delivered. Some use a set jet-size as Alvin Barach did in 1941 with the original entrainment unit, the Mix Mask, and alter the entrainment port size. In this case the lateral pressure created remains constant and the orifice through which air is entrained is changed. The larger the entrainment port the more air that will be entrained, similar to opening a needle valve more, resulting in a lower oxygen percentage.

Humidifiers are not necessary with entrainment devices and may in fact detrimentally affect their performance. Undetected gas leaks or water build up proximal to the jet may alter the delivered oxygen percentage, or the flow of gas to the patient, or both. In addition, the air-to-oxygen ratio is very high for most entrainment ratios used in home care, so the contribution of the oxygen humidifier to the total gas mixture is insignificant. If additional moisture is needed, this is best accomplished by entraining aerosol. Most diluters have a collar-like attachment that facilitates

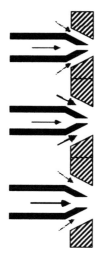

Increased entrainment port size
results in an increased entrainment
of air.

Increased jet size results in
decreased air entrainment.

a.

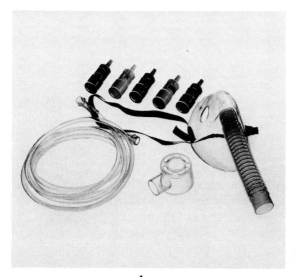

b.

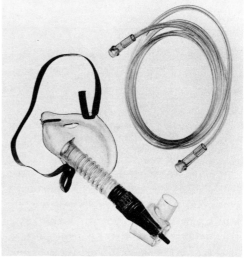

c.

Figure 3.22 A Altering jet size and entrainment port size in entrainment devices.
B Entrainment devices altering jet size. Courtesy of Salter Labs, Arvin, CA. **C** Entrainment
device altering jet size. Courtesy of Salter Labs, Arvin, CA.

Table 3.1 Air: Oxygen Ratios for Common Percentages

$O_2\%$	Air: O_2	Total/L O_2
100	0:1	1.0
70	0.6:1	1.6
60	1:1	2.0
50	1.7:1	2.7
40	3:1	4.0
36	4:1	5.0
34	5:1	6.0
30	8:1	9.0
28	10:1	11.0
26	15:1	16.0
24	25:1	26.0

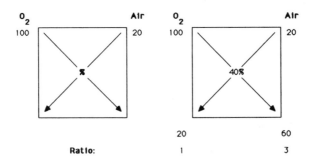

Figure 3.23 Magic box. (Calculates air-to-oxygen ratios.)

entraining aerosol from either a pneumatic nebulizer powered by air or from an ultrasonic nebulizer. It is also important to remember that entrainment devices are very susceptible to resistance. Resistance downstream will be reflected back to the jet and entrainment ports, resulting in a reduction in air entrainment, an increase in the oxygen percentage delivered, and a decrease in the total flow output to the patient. Total flow delivered to the patient from diluters is also crucial. In order for the patient to receive the set oxygen percentage, the diluter must deliver enough flow to meet or exceed his peak inspiratory flow demands. Table 3.1 displays the air oxygen ratios for the common oxygen percentages used in respiratory home care.

If a chart of air/oxygen ratios is not available the "magic box" can be used to approximate the ratios for blending air and oxygen. Figure 3.23 shows the box as it is normally setup with 100% and 20% listed in the upper right and lower right corners, respectively. The percentage of gas that is to have an air/oxygen ratio calculated is placed into the center of the box. In the example on the right, 40% is placed in the center of the box. This percentage (40%) is subtracted from 100%, and 20% is subtracted from 40%. The resulting differences represent the air/oxygen ratios for 40%, which is a 3:1 ratio. Total flow can be determined for any percentage by multiplying the jet flow (as read on the oxygen flowmeter) times both the air and oxygen ratios and adding the two products together.

$$\text{Total Flow} = (\text{Jet Flow} \times \text{Air Ratio}) + (\text{Jet Flow} \times \text{Oxygen Ratio})$$

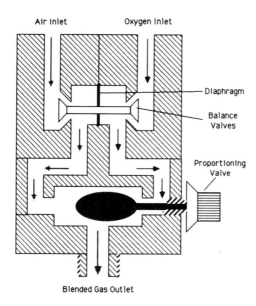

Figure 3.24 Oxygen controller (blender).

As an example, if the jet flow was 10 L/min on a 40% diluter, what would the total flow to the patient be?

Total Flow = (Jet Flow × Air Ratio) + (Jet Flow × Oxygen Ratio)

Total Flow = (10 L/min × 3) + (10 L/min × 1)

Total Flow = 30 L/min + 10 L/min

Total Flow = 40 L/min

As a guide clinically, 30–40 L/min is adequate to meet the peak flows of most adult patients. Another guide that is frequently used is the patient's minute volume times a factor of 4–6 as an approximation of the patient's peak flow. Both numerical values should only be used as guides, and flow should be felt exiting the patient's mask throughout inspiration and if aerosol is being administered, it should be visibly flowing from the exhalation ports throughout inhalation. Table 3.2 demonstrates the comparison of jet flow to total flow at various oxygen percentages.

Safety—As with the oxygen administration devices mentioned previously, all of the safety requirements for administration sites described in chapter 1 apply to entrainment devices.

Oxygen Controllers

Most oxygen percentage controllers (blenders) used in home care require a high pressure source of both air and oxygen. First, the oxygen and air pressure are balanced by a diaphragm and inlet valves for each gas (Figure 3.24). As the pressure of one gas drops lower than the other, the diaphragm moves to the low pressure side, opening the inlet valve more for the lower pressure gas and partially closing the inlet valve for the higher pressure gas. Then the two gases are proportioned or blended by a metering or proportioning valve. The valve acts to open one gas flow as it closes the other. If the oxygen percentage is to be increased, the proportioning valve is rotated to open the oxygen supply more while occluding the air to a greater degree. Most oxygen controllers also have a series of interconnections to provide gas crossover to the opposite source and audible alarms to alert the user in the event of failure of one gas source. Blenders have the advantage of delivering set percentages at pressures up to 50 psig and high flows, which may be required for some respiratory therapy devices such as ventilators and respirators. Blenders are not subject to back pressure and some can be used at lower inlet pressures.

Table 3.2   Comparisons of Jet Flow to Total Flow for Common Oxygen Percentages.

					TOTAL FLOW					
100%	1	2	3	4	5	6	7	8	9	10
70%	1.6	3.2	4.8	6.4	8	9.6	11.2	12.8	14.4	16
60%	2	4	6	8	10	12	14	16	18	20
50%	2.7	5.4	8.1	10.8	13.5	16.2	18.9	21.6	24.3	27
40%	4	8	12	16	20	24	**28**	**32**	**36**	**40**
36%	5	10	15	20	**25**	**30**	35	40	45	50
34%	6	12	18	24	**30**	**36**	42	48	54	60
30%	9	18	**27**	36	45	54	63	72	81	90
28%	11	22	33	44	55	66	77	88	99	110
26%	16	**32**	48	65	80	96	112	128	144	160
24%	**26**	52	78	104	130	156	182	208	234	260
JET FLOW	**1**	**2**	**3**	**4**	**5**	**6**	**7**	**8**	**9**	**10**

(Bold numbers indicate the jet flow required for each oxygen percentage when the patient's peak inspiratory flow requirements are approximately 25L/m.)

					TOTAL FLOW					
100%	1	2	3	4	5	6	7	8	9	10
70%	1.6	3.2	4.8	6.4	8	9.6	11.2	12.8	14.4	16
60%	2	4	6	8	10	12	14	16	18	20
50%	2.7	5.4	8.1	10.8	13.5	16.2	18.9	21.6	24.3	27
40%	4	8	12	16	20	24	28	**32**	**36**	**40**
36%	5	10	15	20	25	**30**	35	40	45	50
34%	6	12	18	24	**30**	**36**	42	48	54	60
30%	9	18	27	**36**	45	54	63	72	81	90
28%	11	22	33	44	55	66	77	88	99	110
26%	16	**32**	48	64	80	96	112	128	144	160
24%	**26**	**52**	**78**	104	130	156	182	208	234	260
JET FLOW	**1**	**2**	**3**	**4**	**5**	**6**	**7**	**8**	**9**	**10**

(Bold numbers indicate the jet flow required for each oxygen percentage when the patient's peak inspiratory flow requirements are approximately 30L/m.)

Table 3.2 *Continued*

				TOTAL	FLOW					
100%	1	2	3	4	5	6	7	8	9	10
70%	1.6	3.2	4.8	6.4	8	9.6	11.2	12.8	14.4	16
60%	2	4	6	8	10	12	14	16	18	20
50%	2.7	5.4	8.1	10.8	13.5	16.2	18.9	21.6	24.3	27
40%	4	8	12	16	20	24	28	32	**36**	**40**
36%	5	10	15	20	25	30	**35**	**40**	**45**	**50**
34%	6	12	18	24	30	**36**	**42**	**48**	**54**	**60**
30%	9	18	27	**36**	**45**	**54**	**63**	**72**	**81**	**90**
28%	11	22	33	**44**	**55**	**66**	**77**	**88**	**99**	**110**
26%	16	32	**48**	**64**	**80**	**96**	**112**	**128**	**144**	**160**
24%	26	52	**78**	**104**	**130**	**156**	**182**	**208**	**234**	**260**
JET FLOW	**1**	**2**	**3**	**4**	**5**	**6**	**7**	**8**	**9**	**10**

(Bold numbers indicate the jet flow required for each oxygen percentage when the patient's peak inspiratory flow requirements are approximately 30L/m.)

Oxygen Analyzers

Virtually all oxygen analyzers used in respiratory home care are one of two types of electrochemical analyzers. The first type is the galvanic fuel cell type. A membrane that is permeable to oxygen covers a hydroxide bath that contains two electrodes (Figure 3.25). As the oxygen combines with the water in the hydroxide bath to form more hydroxyl ions, the negative (usually gold—Au) electrode emits electrons. The negatively charged hydroxyl ions are attracted to the positive electrode (usually made of lead—Pb) and they combine with that electrode forming an oxide and releasing the electrons. The electrons released are measured as current that directly relates to the amount of oxygen diffusing across the membrane and combining with the solution. The amount of oxygen diffusing across the membrane is directly proportional to the partial pressure of oxygen exposed to the membrane, and the meter displays the current as oxygen percentage.

The second type of electrochemical oxygen analyzer uses a polarographic or Clark-type electrode. The polarographic type of electrode works very similar to the galvanic cell. Oxygen diffuses across the membrane and combines with water and electrons at the negative electrode to form more hydroxyl ions (Figure 3.26). The electrodes are charged by current from a battery so that the process is speeded up in a polarographic electrode. The ions flow to the positive (usually silver— Ag) electrode and combine with it forming an oxide on the electrode and releasing electrons. The difference in current between the electrodes is displayed as oxygen percentage.

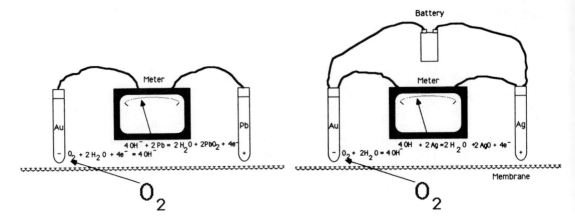

Figure 3.25 Galvanic fuel cell.   **Figure 3.26** Polarographic electrode.

With both the galvanic and polarographic analyzers, the reading is directly related to the partial pressure of oxygen exposed to the membrane, so both are susceptible to changes in barometric pressure such as with changes in altitude. Also, both may be affected by accumulations of water on the membrane surface. Since the polarographic electrode is polarized by a battery, it tends to have a faster response than a galvanic cell; however, galvanic cells tend to last longer. The polarographic type of electrode is most susceptible to marked changes in system pressure on ventilators, although both can be influenced by large changes in pressure above baseline. Recently, oxygen analyzers have been produced that facilitate measuring the percentage of oxygen delivered by concentrators and measuring the concentration of oxygen enclosures. In addition, newer types of fuel cells and polarographic electrodes boast longer sensor life.

Apnea Monitors

Infants that are at risk of sudden infant death syndrome (SIDS) are increasingly being sent home to be monitored. Apnea monitors are used to monitor the infant and provide an alarm in the event that breathing stops. Two types of apnea monitors are commonly used in home respiratory care (Figure 3.27).

The first type monitors electrical impedance of the chest. Since impedance changes as air is drawn into the lungs, this change can be used to detect breathing rate. Electrodes are placed on both sides fo the infant's chest and the monitor displays the respiratory rate and an alarm sounds if the rate drops or ceases. Newer equipment also monitors heart rate and will alarm if bradycardia occurs. Electrode placement is important, and injury has been reported when electrode leads have been connected directly to an electrical outlet.

The second type of apnea monitor uses a grid or pad to monitor the motion of the chest during breathing which in turn, is displayed in the monitor as a breath. If no motion is detected within a certain period of time, the monitor will alarm indicating apnea. Infants that move too much can work their way off of the pad and cause false alarms; however, sand bags placed on either side of the patient may reduce this occurrence.

Parents should be trained in cardio-pulmonary resuscitation (CPR) so they can respond in case prolonged apnea episodes were to occur.

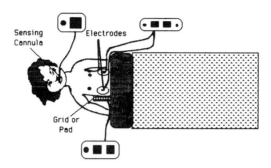

Figure 3.27 Types of Apnea monitors.

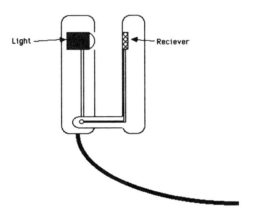

Figure 3.28 Oximeter probe.

Another type of monitoring device has recently been introduced for home respiratory care. The capnograph is being used for measurement of the patient's exhalaed carbon dioxide (CO_2). End-tidal CO_2 recordings are used in analysis of the patient's apneic episodes. The capnograph draws a small sample of exhaled gas into the unit where it is exposed to infrared light. The amount of light absorbed is proportional to the amount of carbon dioxide present in the gas.

Oximeters

Oximeters use a light source and light cell to estimate oxygen saturation of the blood. Different light wave lengths are sent to the probe through fiberoptics, where the light is passed through tissue and the sensor detects the amount of light as an electronic signal (Figure 3.28). The amount of light transmitted through the tissue is constant except for the pulsations of blood being sent through the vessels. The oximeter uses the amount of light passing through the tissue as compared to the amount of light emitted to determine the amount of each wavelength absorbed. The amount of specific light waves that are absorbed has been shown to directly relate to the saturation of the hemoglobin.[13-16] A heater in the probe warms the tissue surface to a temperature of 37–41 degrees C to enhance perfusion to the area.

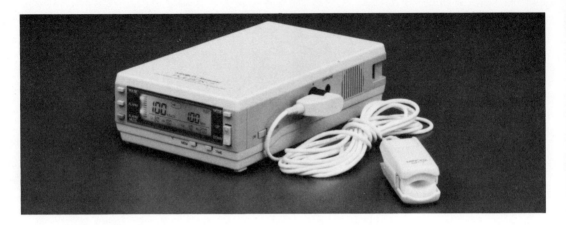

Figure 3.29 Marquest/Minolta Oxymeter. Courtesy of Marquest Medical Products Inc. Englewood, California.

Some oximeter models have a sensor that is attached to the finger (Figure 3.29) as opposed to the ear probe, and another configuration allows attachment to the nasal septum. Pulse rate can also be displayed and is available on most newer models. Oximeters have seen a growing application in home care, because checking patients on home oxygen therapy can be done easily and quickly to determine that their oxygen saturation level is adequate.

Before placing the oximeter probe, one should be certain that the probe is cleaned with isopropyl alcohol (especially the light-emitting and sensing ports). If using the ear piece, rub the ear lobe with isopropyl alcohol for 20–30 seconds to enhance perfusion and to remove oil from the surface of the skin. Place the ear probe so that the light emitter faces toward the skull and be sure that the ear lobe covers the light-emitting and receiving windows. Light from the room will affect the reading. The ear piece should not be placed where there is any cartilage, should be suspended from the ear lobe, and should not be presssing against the side of the head.

When a finger probe is used, the patient should not be wearing fingernail polish or cosmetic fingernails and the nail should be trimmed. The little finger and thumb are not recommended placement sites because coverage of the light ports may not be adequate. The probe should be cleaned with isopropyl alcohol, and you should be sure the light ports are covered completely by the finger.

Oximeters are electrically powered and all precautions described in Chapter 1 for electrical devices used at oxygen administration sites must be observed. Care must be taken, especially in infants, that the probe does not impede circulation distal to the probe placement if the unit is to be left in place for extended periods of time. The probe must be cleaned and disinfected according to the manufacturer's direction, and cannot be immersed or autoclaved. The accuracy of oximeters is affected by the presence of carboxyhemoglobin and jaundice, and alternate methods of assessing oxygenation should be used in those situations.

References

1. McPherson S. P. Respiratory therapy equipment. 3rd ed. St. Louis: CV Mosby Co., 1985.
2. Masferrer R. History of the inhalation therapy-respiratory care profession. In Burton G. G., Hodgkin J. E., eds. Respiratory Care: a guide to clinical practice. 2nd ed. Philadelphia: J. B. Lippincott, 1984.
3. Spearman C. B., Sheldon R. L. Egan's Fundamentals of Respiratory Therapy. 4th ed. St. Louis: CV Mosby Co., 1982.
4. Barach A. Personal communication (unpublished), 1972.
5. National Fire Protection Association: Health care facilities, NFPA No. 99, Boston: National Fire Protection Association, 1984.
6. Redding J. S., McAffe D. D., Parham A. M. Oxygen concentrations received from commonly used delivery systems. South Med J 1978; 71:169.
7. Gibson R. L., et al. Actual tracheal oxygen concentrations with commonly used oxygen equipment. Anesthesiology 1976; 44:71.
8. Lough M. D., Doerschuk C. F. Respiratory therapy. In Lough M. D., Doerschuk C. F., and Stern R. C., eds. Pediatric Respiratory Therapy, 2nd ed. Chicago: Year Book Medical Publishers Inc., 1979.
9. Dawes G. Noise pollution in the neonatal intensive care unit (OF Abstract). Respir Care 1977; 22:424.
10. Chafin T., et al. Noise levels in the neonatal intensive care unit (OF Abstract). Respir Care 1978; 23:64.
11. Hursey F. X. Sound levels generated in a neonatal intensive care unit (OF Abstract). Respir Care 1978; 23:64.
12. Klaus M. H., Fanaroff A. A., eds: Care of the High Risk Neonate. 2nd ed. Philadelphia: Addison-Wesley Publishing Co. Inc, 1979.

4 *Humidifiers and Nebulizers*

Humidity and aerosols are often used in the care of home respiratory patients. Humidity may be needed to make the administration of dry gas comfortable. In patients where their own body's upper airways humidification mechanism is by-passed due to intubation or tracheostomy, humidification is also required.

Aerosols, administered as bland solutions to topically deposit water or saline on the respiratory mucosa, facilitate the removal of secretions. In this application, it is imperative that the patient be well hydrated systemically so that the mucus produced is as thin as possible.[1] Then the addition of liquid to the secretions decreases the viscosity and aids in their removal. Medication nebulizers are also used to deposit pharmacological agents on the airways. If the proper particle size range is selected for depositing specific agents, the local effect of of the medication is maximized and the systemic, undesirable side effects are avoided or minimized.[1]

Devices that are designed to accomplish those objectives will be covered in this chapter, along with methods of modifying the delivery system for improved results.

Simple Humidifiers

There is humidity in the gas that we all breathe normally. The administration of dry gas to respiratory patients at home is made more comfortable with the addition of humidity to the gas. To accomplish this, simple humidifiers have been designed.

Bubble Humidifiers

By far the most common simple humidifier used in home oxygen delivery is the bubble humidifier. A tube directs the incoming gas below the surface of the water (Figure 4.1). It usually passes through some type of diffuser so that the gas breaks up into small bubbles that rise back to the surface of the water. As the gas bubbles pass through the water, they pick up humidity (water vapor). This humidified gas then flows to the outlet, through oxygen connecting tubing, and on to the patient.

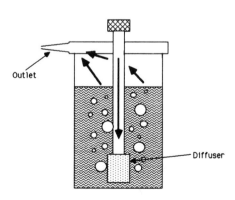

Figure 4.1 Bubble humidifier.

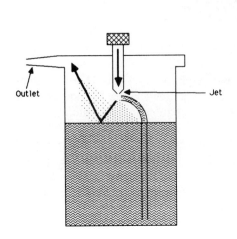

Figure 4.2 Jet humidifier.

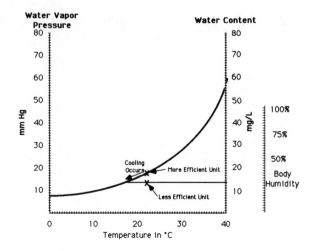

Figure 4.3 Water vapor capacity for simple humidifiers.

Jet Humidifiers

Another type of simple humidifier used in home oxygen therapy is the jet humidifier. This type of humidifier actually produces an aerosol that is *baffled* sufficiently so that the majority of particles evaporate and become humidity. (Baffling is a process where objects are placed in the path of the gas stream which force the stream to make right angles. As a result, the larger particles are split into smaller particles.)

Incoming gas passes through a jet and causes the lateral pressure to drop. Because atmospheric pressure on the surface of the water is higher than the lateral pressure at the jet (Figure 4.2), water is forced up a capillary tube. The gas containing the aerosol particles is directed toward baffles, or obstacles, so that the particles are reduced in size and evaporate. The humidified gas then exits the humidifier outlet and travels to the patient through oxygen connecting tubing.

The debate over which type or brand of humidifier is the "best" can be resolved by considering what happens when humidification occurs. Figure 4.3 displays water vapor pressure and water content of air at various temperatures, as well as the percent of body humidity supplied. When gas flow through a humidifier is initiated, the water in the humidifier is usually at room temperature. As water evaporates to humidify the gas, the water cools. And as this cooling occurs, the gas has a reduced capacity for carrying water. So a humidifier that is very efficient and humidifies gas to nearly 100% relative humidity, cools the water and gas so that the capacity for holding water vapor is lowered. Alternately, a humidifier that does not humidify the gas to as high a relative humidity, also will not cool the gas as much, resulting in a higher capacity. The net result is that both deliver about the same amount of water vapor to the patient.

As mentioned in chapter one, humidifiers must have an audible pressure relief.[2] When selecting a brand of humidifier, it is extremely important to test the audible pop-off for reliability, especially if the unit is to be used at lower flowrates (1 L/min or less). It is also advisable to check the pop-off to be certain that it reseats and that the humidifier itself does not leak around any component connections. This can be accomplished by connecting a high pressure hose from a flowmeter to

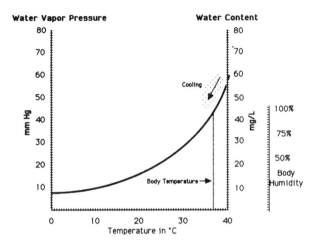

Figure 4.4 Water vapor capacity for heated humidifiers

the humidifier inlet and attaching the oxygen connecting tubing to the outlet, turning the flow-meter on, and then running the humidifier under water in a bucket or tub. Any leaks will be obvious and the connecting tubing can be occluded and then released after the pop-off vents to be sure that it reseats.

Humidifier liquid reservoirs or jars must be made of a clear, transparent material to permit observation of the water level and consistency.[2]

Humidifiers should be cleaned and disinfected at least weekly following the manufacturer's guidelines. Generally, a mild soap is recommended, followed by thorough rinsing. A disinfectant that is not harmful to the plastics is used next, followed by a second thorough rinsing and drying. 0.25% acetic acid can be used as a decontaminating solution.[3] One part white vinegar in three parts water will provide this concentration of acetic acid disinfecting solution. To suppress the growth of bacteria, the use of copper mesh in humidifiers has been reported.[4]

Humidifiers have been shown to emit aerosol particles, probably due to bubble deterioration.[5] However, studies have failed to demonstrate bacteria being transmitted by these particles.[6] Particles that are produced by bubbles breaking up are probably too small to provide a vehicle for bacterial transfer. Nevertheless, humidifiers should be considered and treated as a potential source of contamination.

Heated Humidifiers

Patients whose upper airways have been by-passed due to intubation or tracheotomy may inhale gas at 100% relative humidity at body temperature (body humidity) by using a heated humidifier. In most cases, these humidifiers are heated above body temperature because cooling will occur as gas passes through large diameter tubing on the way to the patient. As this cooling occurs, condensate is produced and collects in the tubing due to the cooled gas having a reduced carrying capacity for humidity (Figure 4.4.) For this reason, the aerosol tubing should angle downward

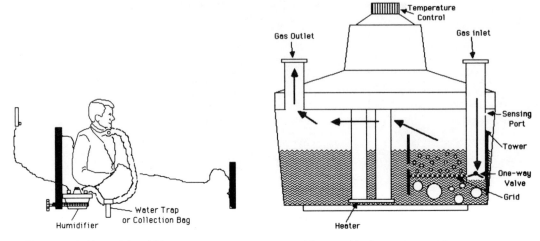

Figure 4.5 Heated humidifier set-up.   **Figure 4.6** Cascade humidifier.

away from the patient so that the condensate drains into the reservoir of the humidifier rather than draining toward the patient (Figure 4.5.) Low spots in the tubing should also be avoided to prevent blockage and water accumulation. Water traps or water collection bags can also be used to collect the condensate if low points in the tubing are unavoidable.

The Bennett Cascade® humidifier in 1966 introduced the concept of an advanced bubble humidifier that is heated (Figure 4.6.) Gas flows down the tower and displaces the heated water in the reservoir over a grid. Gas flows through the grid and into the water above, causing the water to humidify and heat the gas. The heated, humidified gas then exits the outlet port. A one-way valve prevents the back flow of humidified gas, and a small sensing port allows the patient to initiate an assist breath if the Cascade is connected to a ventilator. The temperature of the water is regulated by a thermostatically-controlled heating element, which is sheated in a metal sleeve and suspended in the water. Factors such as the operating temperature, water level in the reservoir, flowrate of gas, room temperature, and length of delivery tubing affect the temperature of the gas reaching the patient. The temperature of the humidified gas should be monitored proximal to the patient connection. Inhaled gas above body temperature can be damaging to the airways in a very short period of time[7]. On the other hand, if the gas is delivered to the patient below body temperature, the water vapor content of the gas can be significantly reduced (Figure 4.4.) In addition, the water in the reservoir can be very hot, so caution should be taken in filling and changing the reservoirs themselves.

More recently Puritan-Bennett released the Cascade II® humidifier, which has a proximal temperature monitoring probe. The probe monitors and displays the temperature of the gas at the patient's airway (Figure 4.7) and the heater adjusts to maintain the temperature that is set by the control. An alarm sounds in the event of disconnection of the probe as an alert to possible inadvertent overheating. Other similar units are available, such as those manufactured by Bear Medical, Ohmeda, and Chemtron.

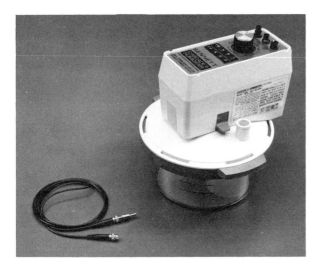

Figure 4.7 Cascade II humidifier. (Compliments of Puritan Bennett.)

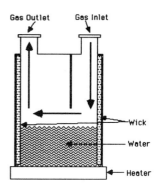

Figure 4.8 Wick-type humidifier.

Wick-Type Humidifier

Another design of heated humidifiers uses a wick that absorbs water by capillary action. Gas comes in contact with the wick where it is heated and humidified. The gas is then directed to the outlet (Figure 4.8.) The Bird 3000 is an example of a pediatric version of a wick-type humidifier. Disposable wick/reservoir models are available also such as the Conchapak from Respiratory Care, Inc., the MR500 from Fisher and Paykel (Isothermal), and the HLC from Travenol. The Vapor-Phase from Inspiron (Cygnus) uses a hydrophobic filter between the water and gas in the chamber allowing only water vapor to pass through.

As mentioned earlier, humidifiers have been shown to emit particles of water, probably from bubble deterioration. The particle size is probably very small and is most likely the reason that bacterial transfer on the droplets has not been shown. However, the condensate will soon make a liquid transfer for the bacteria, and, in the home, these devices should be changed every 24–72 hours.

Heated Wire Circuit

Another adaptation for heated humidifiers is the heated wire circuit. A separate unit controls the heated wires on both the inspiratory and expiratory sides of the circuit. The gas leaves the humidifier at near-body temperature, and the heated wires maintain that temperature through the circuit to the patient. Since the temperature of the gas does not drop appreciably, condensate is eliminated. Heated wire circuits are available from Isothermal and Marquest for infant and adult ventilators.

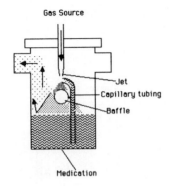

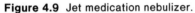

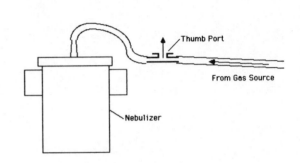

Figure 4.9 Jet medication nebulizer.

Figure 4.10 Nebulizer tee with thumb port in drive line.

Heat and Moisture Exchangers

Heat and moisture exchangers (condensing humidifiers) use a different principle to humidify the inspired gas. These exchangers are placed between the patient and the circuit and when the patient exhales, a hygroscopic material in the filter traps the water vapor and heat from the exhaled breath. During inhalation, the gas is warmed and humidified by the heat and moisture exchanger. Seventy to ninety percent body humidity have been reported with the use of these devices. Companies manufacturing these exchangers are Siemens, Pall, Engstrom, Marquest, Terumo, and AirLife.

Medication Nebulizers

The most common type of simple nebulizer use the Bernoulli's principle to produce an aerosol. The gas passes through a jet, lowering the lateral pressure. As the lateral pressure drops, the atmospheric pressure forces liquid up a small capillary tube. When the liquid hits the gas stream, it breaks up into particles (Figure 4.9.) These particles are then baffled by placing objects (baffles) in their path and forcing the gas stream to make right angles. As a result, the larger particles fall out or are split into smaller particles.

Hand-held Nebulizers

Medication or hand-held nebulizers use this principle. The first nebulizer of this type was introduced in 1938 by the Hudson. Most of the early models incorporated a squeeze bulb to supply gas to the jet or the bulb could be removed and a gas source could be connected. The gas source can power the medication nebulizer continuously until all of the solution is aerosolized or a tee with a thumb port can be added in the supply line (Figure 4.10.) The patient is instructed to occlude the port in the tee with his thumb just before inhaling and then to release his thumb from the port when exhalation begins.

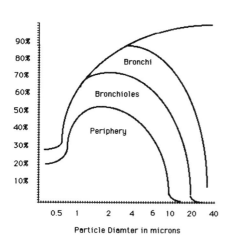

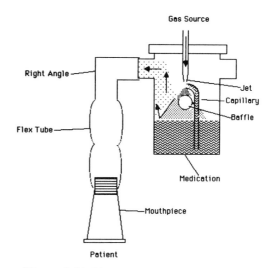

Figure 4.11 Aerosol particle deposition. (Modified from Cushing IE and M. Miller WF. Nebulization therapy. In Safar P, Editor: Respiratory Therapy, Philadelphia: FA Davis Co., 1965.)

Figure 4.12 Medication nebulizer set-up for small particle delivery.

The patient should be instructed to breath slowly through an open mouth and to take a deep breath (1200–1400 ml or 1 1/2–2 times his normal tidal volume) and then hold it at the end of inspiration (up to 15 seconds or as long as he can tolerate).[1,2] This method provides the best penetration and deposition of aerosol. Furthermore, it can be predicted where in the tracheobronchial tree the majority of the aerosol particles will be deposited (Figure 4.11.) It is desirable to select particle size to produce optimum penetration and to avoid side effects. The larger the particle, the more solution is deposited with each droplet. If bland solution is being delivered, a particle size that deposits the most volume of solution can be selected. However, if the medication being aerosolized is a potent pharmacological agent, such as a bronchodilator, a smaller particle size should be selected so that the highest percentage of particles reach the targeted area of the respiratory tract. Undesirable systemic side effects are caused when particles are deposited on the upper airways, so large particles must be avoided when delivering potent agents. As an example, a particle range of 3–5 microns will deposit the largest *number* of particles at the bronchiole level, while minimizing systemic side effects if a bronchodilator is being delivered. A particle size of 8–20 microns will deposit the largest *volume* of solution at the bronchioles if a bland mixture is being administered. In fact, potent bronchodialators have been administered with maximum topical effects and minimum systemic side effects when submicronic aerosols were used.[8] Figure 4.12 demonstrates a nebulizer set-up for delivering small particles. The right angle and aerosol tubing provide additional baffling and the reservoir tubing allows for the accumulation of small particles during the expiratory phase to be available for the next inspiration. Water is also the best solution for diluting bronchodilators because it will reduce the solute/solvent content of these large molecular structure solutions so that they will not act hygroscopic and grow upon entering the respiratory tract.[8]

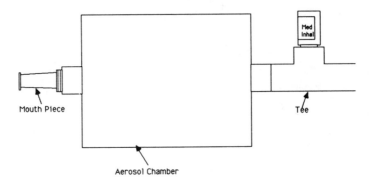

Figure 4.13 Aerosol chamber.

Unit Dose Inhalers

Unit dose inhalers are also used for the delivery of certain medications. Recently, devices have been released to aid in improving the particle penetration and deposition with this method of aerosol administration. In the unit dose inhaler, medication is delivered into the aerosol chamber (Figure 4.13) and the patient breathes from the chamber through a mouthpiece. These chambers aid in reducing the deposit of particles against the back of the throat and also allows the larger particles to drop out before they are inhaled. These devices can be helpful for patients who have trouble coordinating inspiration to discharge the medication, such as with pediatric patients. Aerosol chambers are available from Hudson, Key Pharmaceuticals, & Monaghan.

Medication nebulizers and associated devices should be rinsed off with water and dried between treatments. They should be cleaned daily in a mild soap, rinsed, disinfected, rinsed again, and dried according to the recommendations of the manufacturer or supplier.

Entrainment Nebulizers

Larger volume jet nebulizers are designed for continuous use and usually have air entrainment oxygen percentage control capabilities. These nebulizers also use the Bernoulli's principle to nebulize the liquid, and to entrain air to deliver set oxygen concentrations. The jet size is fixed and the port size is varied to change the amount of air entrained and, therefore, the oxygen concentration delivered (Figure 4.14.)

As mentioned in chapter 3, the total flow to the patient must meet or exceed his peak inspiratory flow demands. 40 L/min is generally considered an average peak flow for the purposes of initially setting-up the aerosol. Once the aerosol in placed on the patient, there should be aerosol visibly flowing from the exhalation ports throughout inspiration to be assured that the total flow to the patient exceeds the inhalation requirements. In patients who have lower minute volumes, during inspiration the jet flow can be reduced until the flow of aerosol seen through the exhalation ports vanishes and then increase the jet flow until aerosol is again visible throughout inspiration. This method should also be used when maximum aerosol density is desirable. In other words, the higher the total flow the lower the aerosol density. Air/oxygen entrainment ratios and calculation of those

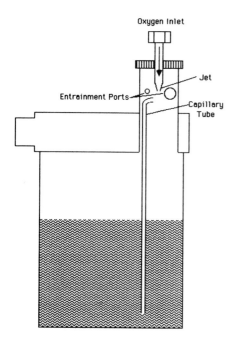

Figure 4.14 Entrainment nebulizer.

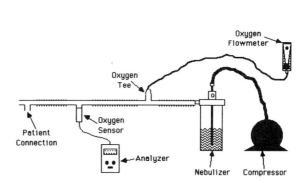

Figure 4.15 Oxygen addition to a nebulizer powered by compressed air.

ratios is covered in chapter 3. If the total flow is too low, air will be drawn in during inspiration and the percentage of oxygen reaching the patient will drop. Figure 4.15 displays the jet flows required at various oxygen percentages to deliver a total flow of 40 L/min to the patient.

Solutions used in pneumatic jet nebulizers are bland, usually water or saline. Normal saline, being isotonic, is the least irritating, but it may tend to pool in the lungs of small children and non-mobile patients. Water will not pool, but is the more irritating and results in the highest increase in airways resistance. Half normal saline (0.45%) has been used as a compromise. It is not as irritating as water and does have an osmotic gradient to prevent pooling. As mentioned previously, the reservoir should be transparent so that the liquid level is easily observed.

Currently, the lowest oxygen percentage setting available on pneumatic nebulizers is 28%, with some units having 35 or 40% as their lowest setting. When oxygen percentages below the lowest setting are required, there are two methods of setting the nebulizer up to accomplish this.

The first method is to power the nebulizer with air and bleed in oxygen (Figure 4.15.) This requires an oxygen analyzer to measure the oxygen bleed flow until the desired F_IO_2 is reached.

The second method employs an entrainment device (diluter.) The diluter supplies the patient with the set oxygen percentage and the aerosol is supplied from a pneumatic nebulizer powered by air from a small air compressor. An aerosol collar is placed over the entrainment ports of the diluter (Figure 4.16) which entrains the aerosol from the air driven nebulizer. Another version of this approach is to use an air entrainment device to deliver the aerosol produced by an ultrasonic nebulizer (Figure 4.17.)

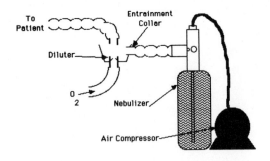

Figure 4.16 Low oxygen percentage aerosol delivery.

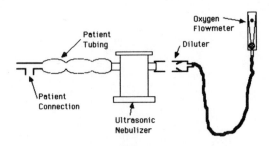

Figure 4.17 Ultrasonic nebulizer with an oxygen diluter.

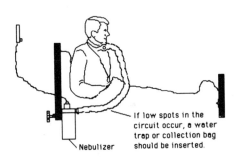

Figure 4.18 Circuit set-up for drainage of rain-out.

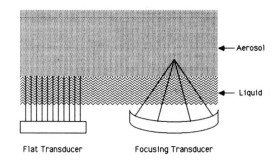

Figure 4.19 Ultrasonic transducers.

Nebulizers and other equipment that make up the patient circuit should be cleaned with a mild soap, rinsed, disinfected with an appropriate solution as recommended by the manufacturer, rinsed again, and dried every 24–72 hours. If disposable, the equipment should discarded. Nebulizing 10 cc of 0.25% acetic acid has also been shown to be effective in decontaminating nebulizers.[3]

Care must be taken with heaters to ensure proper grounding. Otherwise the nebulizer solution can create a grounding pathway to the patient due to condensate. Heaters should be turned off when flow to the nebulizer is stopped to prevent injury to the patient from overheating of the water in the reservoir. The temperature of the delivered aerosol should always be monitored proximal to the patient because high temperature aerosols can damage the airways in a short period of time.[9]

Particle "rain-out," especially in heated aerosols must be controlled. The tubing should slope downward, away from the patient, or water traps or collection bags should be used (Figure 4.18). Low spots in the tubing should be avoided as rain-out may accumulate sufficiently to alter the oxygen percentage or the flow of gas may send a bolus of water to the patients airway.

Ultrasonic Nebulizers

Ultrasonic nebulizers are designed with a piezoelectric transducer. A piezoelectric transducer can expand and contract as current isapplied intermittently. This causes the transducer to vibrate and to produce ultrasonic waves, which are directed toward the surface of the water (Figure 4.19.)

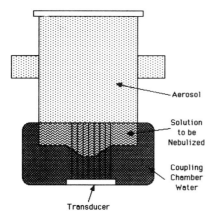

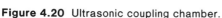

Figure 4.20 Ultrasonic coupling chamber.

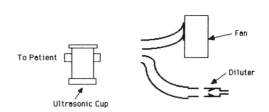

Figure 4.21 Ultrasonic nebulizer with a fan or diluter.

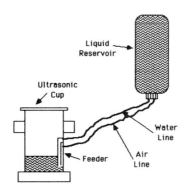

Figure 4.22 Continuous feed system for an ultrasonic nebulizer.

When the ultrasonic waves hit the surface of the water, aerosol is produced. Transducers can be flat and direct the ultrasonic waves straight upward, or they can be curved so the the waves are focused at or slightly above the surface of the water. Generally, curved transducers have a higher output range than the flat type. The material used in the transducer is fragile, and, when cleaning the unit, care must be taken to avoid causing damage. Some ultrasonics nebulizers have a shielded transducer, where a piece of metal is bonded to the transducer itself to protect it from damage.

A certain amount of heat results from the expansion and contraction of the transducer. To disperse this heat, a coupling chamber is filled with water (Figure 4.20.) The solution to be nebulized is contained in a cup that is separated from the coupling chamber by a thin transparent diaphragm. A fan or entrainment device is usually employed to deliver the aerosol to the patient through large bore tubing (Figure 4.21.) A continuous feed system patterned after a chicken feeder can also be added for continuous aerosol delivery (Figure 4.22.)

Ultrasonic nebulizers have a fairly small particle range of about 1–10 microns and a mean particle size of around 3 microns. Compared to pneumatic nebulizers, the ultrasonics have a considerably higher output. Some units are capable of delivering as high as 6 ml/minute. For this reason higher output levels should be used with caution in infants and immobile patients. As mentioned earlier, saline tends to pool and water is very irritating, so 0.45 saline may be preferred, especially in these patients.

Ultrasonic nebulizers are electric powered and their use must comply with all safety requirements of electrical devices used at the site of oxygen administration outlined in chapter 1. Severe damage can occur if a finger contacts the surface or focal point of the ultrasonic waves. The unit should be turned off while working with either the ultrasonic cup or the coupling compartment.

Room Humidifiers

Recently, ultrasonic "humidifiers" have been introduced. In actuality, they are ultrasonic nebulizers which produce aerosol into the room. The aerosol evaporates and humidifies the room, hence the name "humidifier".

Another type of room humidifier that has been in use for many years is the centrifugal nebulizers. A spinning disc rotates and turns the hollow shaft that draws water up to the disc, much like an auger. Once the water reaches the surface of the spinning disc, it is thrown outward due to centrifugal force through breaker combs, which break the water up into particles forming an aerosol. Air from fan blades send the aerosol into the room where it evaporates.

Room humidifiers have been difficult to clean because they did not disassemble easily, the motor could not be immersed, and the reservoir volume is too largely to be totally immersed. Newer units have disposable or removable chambers and the ultrasonic type are also easier to clean.

Again, room humidifiers are electrically powered and must be used in accordance with the safety regulations described in chapter 1.

References

1. Miller W. F. Fundamental principles of aerosol therapy. Resp Care 1972; 17:295.
2. Miller W. F. Aerosol therapy in acute and chronic respiratory disease. Arch Intern Med 1973; 131:148.
3. National Fire Protection Association: Health care facilities, NFPA No. 99, Boston: National Fire Protection Association, 1984.
4. Masferrer R., DuPriest M. Six year evaluation of decontamination of respiratory therapy equipment. Resp Care 1977; 22:145.
5. Nelson E. J. Respiratory therapy equipment contamination survelliance program—Part I, Series 5. Seattle: Olympic Medical Corp.
6. Schulze T., Edmondson E.B., Pierce A.K., et al: Studies of a new humidifying device as a potential source of bacterial aerosols. Amer Rev Resp Dis 96:517–519, 1967.
7. Vesley D., et al. Bacterial output from three respiratory therapy humidifying devices. Resp Care 1979; 24:228.
8. Miller W. F. Personal communication, 1975.
9. Miller W. F. Fundamental principles of aerosol therapy. Resp Care 1972; 17:295.

5 *Artificial Airways and Resuscitators*

Management of the airway is a critical facet of the care for the respiratory home patient. As the number of patients who are being discharged from hospitals increases, so does the number of patients sent home on ventilators. Therefore, the frequency of home care practitioners managing artificial airways will also increases. Patients may also require an artificial airway following discharge from laryngectomy or may require improved airway access for suctioning.

Airways

Nasopharyngeal Airways

Nasopharyngeal airways are frequently used to reduce upper airway obstruction caused by the tongue while patients sleep. These devices have also been shown to facilitate suctioning.[1] Nasopharyngeal airways, rather than oral airways, are generally better tolerated in patients who are awake. The nasal airway is designed to be inserted into the nose and directed posteriorly, following the curvature of the nasopharynx. The tip of the nasopharyngeal airway should be just above the epiglottis to hold the tongue anteriorly and allow a clear passage for air flow (Figure 5.1). If the airway is inserted too far, the tip may force the epiglottis downward, occluding the entrance into the larynx. If the airway is not long enough, it may actually force the base of the tongue downward and contribute to upper airway obstruction. The appropriate length of the nasopharyngeal airway can be approximated as the distance from the tip of the patient's nose to the meatus (opening) of the ear.[1]

Nasal airways have a large flange at the nasal end to discourage it from traveling further inward. If the flange appears too small in relation to the patient's nares, a large safety pin can be placed off-center through the flange as an additional safeguard.[3]

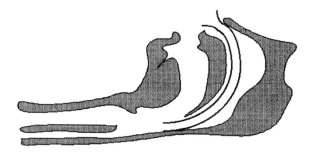

Figure 5.1 Nasal airway.

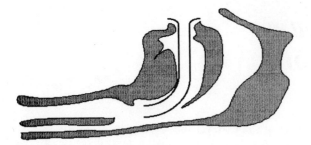

Figure 5.2 Oral airway.

Figure 5.3 Elevation of the chin and extension of the neck.

Nasal airways should be completely lubricated with petroleum jelly or a water soluble lubricant before being inserted. Excessive petroleum jelly should not be used or it will migrate into the patient's airways; however, the jelly aids in the later removal of the airway more effectively than water soluble lubricants.

The airway should be gently introduced and directed posteriorly through the nasal passage. It should never be forced if resistance is encountered. If a nasal airway will be left in for long periods of time, it should be removed and another placed in the opposite nare every 24–48 hours.[3]

Nasal airways are not intended for emergency ventilation, but if the mouth and other nare are occluded, short term gas delivery can be attempted in the airway until intubation is performed. The effective administration of aerosols is compromised through a nasal airway, and the mouth is still the preferred route.

Oropharyngeal Airways

Oropharyngeal airways are more quickly and easily inserted when the need arises. However, an oral airway should not be inserted into a conscious patient or gagging, vomiting, or laryngospasm may result.[1]

The oral airway is generally inserted into the mouth from one side and then twisted into place so that the posterior tip is moved into position behind the base of the tongue, just above the epiglottis (Figure 5.2). Length is as important in an oral airway as with a nasal airway. If the airway is too long, it may push the epiglottis downward occluding the opening to the larynx and if it is too short, the airway may push the base of the tongue downward causing obstruction. The oral end of the airway should be rigid to prevent the patient from occluding the opening by biting down. Most oral airways incorporate a flange to minimize migration further into the pharynx.

A maneuver that may aid in the insertion of an airway is extension of the neck and elevation of the chin into the "sniffing position" (Figure 5.3). This measure is also generally effective when upper airway obstruction is caused by the tongue.

Oropharyngeal airways are generally of two primary designs.[4] The Guedel type has a hollow passage for pharyngeal suctioning while the Berman type has an I-beam construction that allows passage of the suction catheter down either side. Figures 5.4A and 5.4B show some common variations to these two basic types of oral airways.

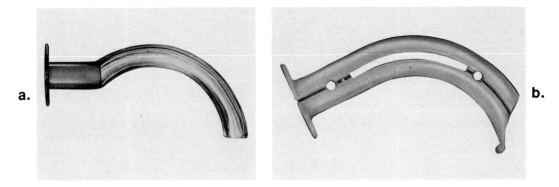

Figure 5.4A and B Oral airways. Courtesy of Hudson Oxygen Therapy Sales Company, Temecula, CA.

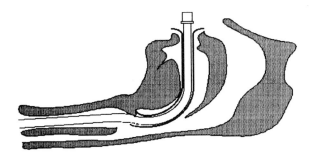

Figure 5.5 Berman intubating airway.

The Berman intubating airway, introduced by the Hudson Oxygen Company, is reported to facilitate blind oral intubation (Figure 5.5).[5] The airway is designed so that the posterior tip rests just above the epiglottis, and angles anteriorly helping to guide the endotracheal tube into the larynx. Once the endotracheal tube is in place, the airway can be separated into two halves that can be removed, leaving the tube in place.

Esophageal Obturator Airway

The esophageal obturator airway is designed to place a cuffed tube into the esophagus (Figure 5.6). The cuffed end of the tube is closed. Once the obturator is inserted, the cuff is inflated to seal the esophagus. The upper portion of the tube has a face mask which seals the patient's mouth and nose. Gas that is introduced into the unit passes through the ventilation ports in the upper portion of the obturator and into the patient's airways. The mask can be removed once the patient resumes spontaneous breathing, but the esophageal cuff should not be deflated until the patient is alert and suction capabilities are present to manage any vomiting that will likely occur.

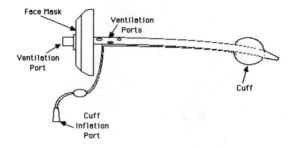

Figure 5.6 Esophageal obturator airway.

The esophageal gastric tube airway is a modification of the original obturator airway design, which facilitates the decompression of the stomach with a gastric tube prior to deflating the esophageal cuff. This reduces the chance of the patient aspirating vomitus. Ventilation is accomplished directly into the mask from the airway port. Esophageal obturators are available in one adult size.

Problems that have been reported with the esophageal obturator airway include esophageal perforation from over-inflation of the cuff, inadvertent tracheal intubation, gastric distention, vomiting and aspiration upon removal of the tube, and laceration of the esophagus from either traumatic insertion or removal with the cuff inflated.[3]

Endotracheal Tubes

Design of Endotracheal Tubes

Endotracheal tubes provide the most common form of artificial airway. The airway is usually established through the mouth with an oral endotracheal tube, especially in an emergency, but it can be placed nasally (with a nasal tracheal tube). Establishing an artificial airway relieves airway obstruction, protects the airway from aspiration, facilitates suctioning, and enhances mechanical ventilation.[1] On the other hand, the use of an artificial airway bypasses the normal humidification mechanism of the body, the normal defense against bacterial invasion, and the normal ability to communicate, and it interferes with the patient's ability to cough. It is vital that the endotracheal tube be positioned correctly, or the artificial airway can compromise the patient even further than his own inadequate airway. If the tube is inserted into the esophagus, ventilation will not take place, and if inserted too far into the airway, only the right lung may be ventilated.

Virtually all endotracheal tubes in use today have a permanently attached cuff, except for the smaller uncuffed pediatric tubes (Figure 5.7). When properly inserted, the cuff rests in the trachea, between the larynx and the carina to provide a seal for positive pressure ventilation. The cuff also prevents secretions in the pharynx from migrating into the trachea. Tubes used in children are not cuffed because of the small diameter of the upper airway. The largest size tube is inserted to facilitate ventilation, leaving little or no room for a cuff. The Cole tube is designed with a taper to a smaller diameter at the tip which then seals the airway in pediatric patients at the cricoid, the smallest passageway in a child's airway.

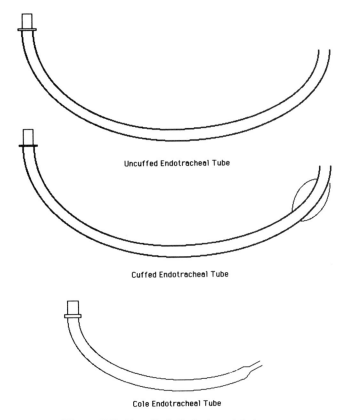

Uncuffed Endotracheal Tube

Cuffed Endotracheal Tube

Cole Endotracheal Tube

Figure 5.7 Uncuffed, Cuffed, and Cole-type endotracheal tubes.

Cuff Pressure

Modern endotracheal tubes use a high-residual volume, low-pressure cuff as compared to the low-residual volume, high-pressure cuffs of the past. The newer versions are cylindrical-shaped as opposed to the spherical shape of high pressure cuffs (Figure 5.8). The high-pressure cuffs were capable of generating pressures of as high as 300 mm Hg against the walls of the trachea. The low pressure cuffs may be capable of exerting pressures of less than 25 mm Hg.[4] Since the intra-arterial pressure in the adult trachea is approximately 30 mm Hg pressure and the venous end of the capillary bed is approximately 18 mm Hg pressure, ideal cuff pressure should be below these values so as not to impede or stop blood flow to the tracheal mucosa in the area of the pressurized cuff. In fact pressures in excess of 5 mm Hg will stop lymphatic flow, resulting in mucosa edema.[1] High pressure cuffs can cause tracheal wall damage within a very short period of time and have no place in modern respiratory care.

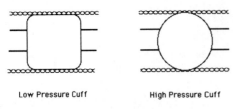

Low Pressure Cuff   High Pressure Cuff

Figure 5.8 Low and high pressure cuffs.

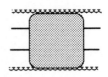

Figure 5.9 Kamen-Wilkinson Fome Cuf.

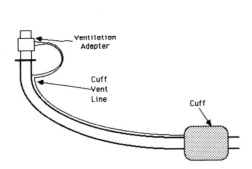

Figure 5.10 Ventilation adapter for the Fome Cuf.

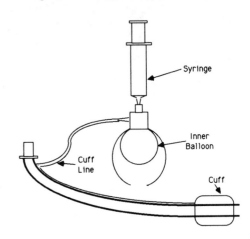

Figure 5.11 McGinnis Balloon.

One attempt at limiting cuff pressure against the tracheal wall is the Kamen-Wilkinson Fome Cuf by Bivona (Figure 5.9). The silicone cuff is filled with polyurethane foam. The foam within the cuff is deflated by removing air prior to being inserted and then is allowed to regain its shape when placed in the trachea. This design maintains a pressure against the tracheal wall of approximately 20 mm Hg if used properly.[4]

Using the proper size is important. If the tube is too small, a proper seal will not be attained and if the tube and cuff are too large, a pressure of greater than 20 mm Hg will be exerted on the tracheal wall.[6]

A ventilation adapter is available that provides a "communication" from the patient airway to the cuff. The pressure applied during inspiration is transmitted to the cuff and is helpful in maintaining a seal at higher ventilation and/or PEEP pressures (Figure 5.10). The manufacturer recommends deflation at least daily to assess the integrity of the cuff and to prevent it from adhering to the tracheal wall.

Another approach to limiting the cuff pressure is the use of a pressure-limiting device. The McGinnis balloon was the first device of this type and is incorporated on the Lanz and Extracorporeal tubes. The inner balloon limits the pressure due to its elasticity to 16–18 mm Hg pressure (Figure 5.11) unless it is expanded to the size of the outer protective sheath.[4] As much as 200 cc of air can be injected without the balloon approaching the size of the outer balloon.[4] A pressure valve prevents the flow of gas back into the balloon during a pressurized breath.

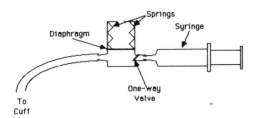

Figure 5.12 Spring-loaded cuff, pressure-limiting device.

Spring-loaded devices to limit cuff pressure are available on the Shiley tracheostomy tube and as a separate device from Respironics (Figure 5.12). Both devices limit the cuff pressure to about 25 mm Hg pressure. The Respironics has the capability of being teed into the patient circuit for patients on higher levels of PEEP so that the 25 mm Hg limit occurs above PEEP pressure.

Complications and Care

The complications of endotracheal intubation include bypassing the normal humidification and bacterial defense mechanisms of the tracheobronchial tree. The most common problems associated with the use of artificial airways relate to those compromises. The need for heated humidification cannot be over-emphasized in the care of long-term ventilator patients.

Aseptic technique must be followed when working with all patients who have artificial airways, especially those with heated humidification systems on ventilators. The patient's ability to effectively cough is removed and suctioning must replace the natural method of secretion removal. This adds greatly to the potential for bacterial contamination, thus it is imperative that sterile technique be used when suctioning. The respiratory care practitioner must be very aware of what complications can occur. The patient loses his ability to communicate so one must make extra effort in communicating with the patient. The adequacy of ventilation must be assessed frequently. The practitioner must be certain that the tube has not slipped into the right main stem bronchus and that both lungs are being ventilated. Again, proper humidification is imperative to prevent secretions from building up and partially occluding the tube. It is important that the chest be auscultated to be certain that the lungs are being ventilated equally.

Materials used for endotracheal, as well as tracheostomy tubes, must meet the standards of the Z-79 Committee of the American National Standards Institute (ANSI). The "I.T." symbol on the tube indicates that the material used in its construction has been implant-tested for tissue reactivity. Other markings on the tube include the name of the manufacturer, whether the tube is an oral or nasal tube, the inside (I.D.) and outside (O.D.) diameter, and the length of the tube in centimeters.

If tubes are resterilized, care must be taken to assure removal of all residual toxins prior to reuse. They must aerated properly if ethylene oxide sterilization is used, or rinsed thoroughly if using chemical solutions decontamination. Tubes that have been sterilized by gamma radiation should not be resterilized with ethylene oxide as toxic levels of ethylene chlorohydrin have been reported.[7] Tubes that are intended for single patient use should be considered disposable and not resterilized.

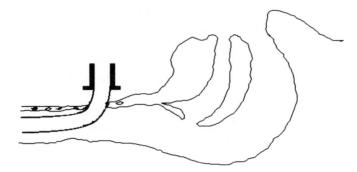

Figure 5.13 Tracheostomy tube.

Tracheostomy Tubes

Design and Pressures

Most patients being mechanically ventilated in the home will have a tracheostomy tube in place, rather than an endotracheal tube. The insertion of a tracheostomy tube is standard for long-term mechanical ventilation and airway management because the upper airway and glottis is bypassed. The tracheostomy tube is placed through the incision in the throat (Figure 5.13). The same principle as those described for cuffs on endotracheal tubes applies for cuffs on tracheostomy tubes. The high-residual volume low-pressure cuffs, the Fome Cuf, and pressure-regulating devices are available for tracheostomy tubes also. Patients have been managed with an endotracheal tube in place for as long as six weeks, but laryngeal lesions are a real possibility.[1] In addition, patients with tracheostomy tubes are easier to stabilize, suctioning is facilitated, and the patient can eat. The tracheostomy tube is also better tolerated by the patient for long periods of time. Generally, adult patients have a tracheostomy tube placed within 7–10 days or in children with uncuffed endotracheal tubes within 2–3 weeks.[3]

Complications and Care

Immediate complications of tracheostomy placement include bleeding, pneumothorax, air embolism, subcutaneous, and mediastinal emphysema. Complications that occur later and that are more likely encountered in home care include infection, hemorrhage, airway obstruction, swallowing dysfunction, and tracheoesophageal fistula[1]. Infection is an ever-present concern with tracheostomy and endotracheal tubes, because the upper airway is bypassed. The respiratory care practitioner must be alert to fever and auscultatory changes that might suggest increased pulmonary infiltrate. Bleeding may occur from the tracheostomy site or tracheal wall. Massive hemorrhage can occur from erosion or from the tube intrusion into the innominate artery. Over-distended cuffs or detachable cuffs that slip over the end of the tube, as well as kinking of the tube itself, can be the cause of obstruction. Normal swallowing may be disturbed when the trachea is secured to the neck via the tracheostomy tube, but this situation usually disappears when the tube is removed.[1] The occurrence of a tracheoesophageal fistula is caused by the pressure of the cuff and tube on the tracheal wall resulting in tracheal ischemia. The importance of low-pressure cuffs, minimum occlusion volumes in inflating the cuff, and monitoring cuff pressures cannot be over-emphasized. Also imperative is the use of proper humidification in the long term care of patients on ventilators with artificial airways.

The tracheostomy tube should be properly secured with ties and a minimum of traction should exist from tubings connected to it. A replacement tube should be kept on hand at all times in the event that the tube is accidentally removed. The site should be cleaned with 3% hydrogen peroxide, rinsed with sterile saline, and a new dressing applied on a routine basis, frequent enough to keep the incision dry and free of secretions.[1] With proper humidification techniques, it has been suggested that tubes need not be replaced on a routine basis as long as they are functioning properly, and there is not an infectious process in the airway or at the wound site.[1] Others have suggested that tracheostomy tube be changed at least weekly.[8]

Since the patient's normal cough mechanism is bypassed with an artificial airway, suctioning is a vital function of the respiratory home care practitioner.

Acute hypoxemia is the most common side effect of suctioning. Patients who have artificial airways in place are frequently on elevated inspired oxygen levels. Suctioning interrupts that oxygen level. Frequently, acute hypoxemia secondary to suctioning causes heart rate and/or rhythm abnormalities. In adults, tachycardia will most often be seen as the initial signal, while pediatric patients will more likely display bradycardia.[1] Any significant change in heart rate or rhythm during suctioning should be attributed to the procedure and ventilation and oxygenation should be re-established without delay. Pre-oxygenating the patient with larger than tidal volume breaths, as well as providing an oxygen-enriched atmosphere around the catheter to prevent room air from entering the airways has been shown to be helpful in avoiding hypoxemia.[1]

Hypotension may also occur due to bradycardia secondary to vagal stimulation, or from direct stimulation of the trachea resulting in prolonged paroxysmal coughs.[1] Hypotension along with hypoxemia and arrhythmias are best avoided with proper suctioning technique, which includes pre-oxygenation, suctioning limited to 10 seconds, and close cardiac monitoring.[1] Lung collapse from using a catheter that is too large to enable air to be drawn in around it has been reported.[9] A good rule of thumb is to use a suction catheter that is smaller than one half the internal diameter of the tube.[1]

Mucosal damage occurs during the suctioning process, and minimizing the severity should be foremost in the practitioner's mind. The appropriate vacuum level, that is enough to adequately remove secretions but no more, generally occurs in the range of -80 to -120 mm Hg pressure. The use of catheters with a ring tip to minimize the catheter's side ports from adhering to the mucosa when suction is applied is considered to be of value by some authors.[1] Suction should be applied only when the catheter is stationary in the airway. Applying suction while moving the catheter in or out of the airway causes increased mucosal damage. Sterile technique must always be followed to minimize contamination. A new, sterile catheter should be used for each suctioning procedure and the hand that manipulates the catheter must be covered by a sterile glove. The appropriate method of suctioning an artificial airway is described below.[1]

1. Pre-oxygenate and hyperinflate the patient for several breaths prior to suctioning. In the home, this is most frequently accomplished with a manual resuscitator capable of delivering 100% oxygen.

2. Insert the catheter without applying suction until the tip is approximately at the level of the carina. A slight obstruction may be felt, and the catheter should be withdrawn a short distance. Then intermittent suction should be applied as the catheter is is rotated. Using intermittent suctioning and rotating the catheter help to minimize mucosal damage.
3. Do not leave the catheter in the airway for longer than 10–15 seconds. The time that the patient is off ventilatory support and oxygenation should not be longer than 20 seconds. Observe the patient and the cardiac monitor. If there is any sign of significant heart rate or rhythm change, stop the suctioning procedure and hyperinflate the patient with 100% oxygen.
4. Re-oxygenate and hyperinflate the patient for at least five deep breaths and return the patient to the ventilator with the settings established prior to suctioning. Be certain that the patient's vital signs have returned to baseline values if it is necessary to suction again. Then use a new, sterile catheter and glove and repeat the steps above. Following tracheal suctioning, the same catheter can be used for oropharyngeal suctioning but must not be reintoduced into the trachea. Suctioning should be initiated when there is clinical evidence of secretions present in the trachea and should not be performed routinely. This will minimize mucosal damage.

Tracheostomy tubes must comply with the Z-79 standards described for endotracheal tubes and the same cleaning and sterilizing considerations apply.

Fenestrated Tracheostomy Tubes

The fenestrated tracheostomy tube allows the patient to breath around the tube and through the fenestration or port if the inner cannula is removed and the cuff is deflated. This allows the patient to speak and provides the practitioner an opportunity to assess the patient's ability to breath on his own before removing the tube. However, the resistance though the fenestration and around the tube may be significantly higher than the patient would experience without the tube in place.

The Pitt Speaking Tracheostomy Tube has a small tube which opens above the cuff and is connected to a gas flow of 4–6 L/min through a wye. When the patient occludes the open port of the wye, the gas flow is directed through the vocal cords. The cuff must be inflated for speech to occur.

One-way valve units are also available that are attached to the tracheostomy tube, but the cuff must be deflated. The patient draws gas in through the one-way valve and then must exhale through the vocal cords. Examples of these devices include the Passy-Muir tracheostomy speaking valve and the Trach-Talk from Olympic.

Tracheostomy buttons can be placed into the stoma to keep it patent and allow suctioning (Figure 5.14). The Olympic trach button and the Kistner button are examples of this type of device. The Olympic unit has spacers to adjust the position of the tube in the trachea and has an inner cannula. The Kistner button has a removable one-way valve attachment.

An electronic device is available from Dacomed called the CyberSet. When activated by a button, the main unit generates a tone and directs a flow of gas through a tube that exits above the cuff of the endotracheal tube (Figure 5.15). As the gas flows through the patient's mouth, the patient must form words from the tone.

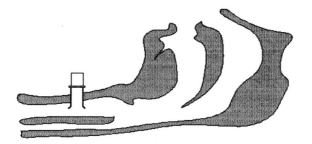

Figure 5.14 Tracheostomy button.

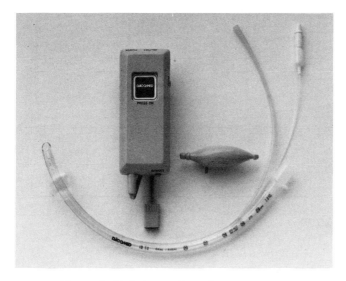

Figure 5.15 Cyberset Tone Generator and tube.

Manual Resuscitator

Self-inflating manual resuscitators provide the capability of manually ventilating the patient in the event of an arrest, power or equipment failure, and for pre-oxygenating and hyperinflating the patient before and after suctioning. A manual resuscitator should be kept at the patient's bedside if he is considered to be at risk of respiratory arrest or if the patient is being mechanically ventilated.

Manual resuscitators are generally constructed with one of two types of nonrebreathing valves.[4] The first type of valve is the spring loaded valve (Figure 5.16). When the bag is compressed to ventilate the patient, the gas flows from the bag, pushing the ball or disc upward, thus compressing the spring and occluding the exhalation port. Gas from the bag is then directed to the patient's

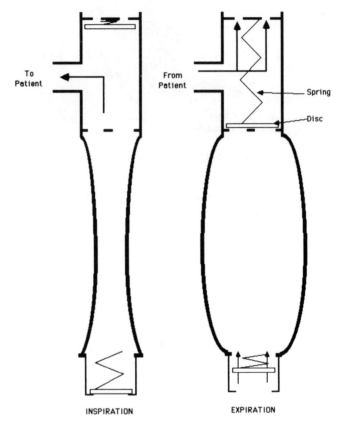

To Patient

From Patient

Spring

Disc

INSPIRATION

EXPIRATION

Figure 5.16 Spring/disc resuscitator valve.

airways. When the bag is released, the spring forces the ball/disc back against the bag outlet and the patient's exhalation occurs passively through the exhalation ports and the bag refills through the bag inlet one-way valve. Examples of this type of manual resuscitator are the Ohio (Ohmeda) Hope and Hope II, the original AMBU, the Air Viva, and the Stat Blue disposable manual resuscitator by Vital Signs.

The second type of valve is the diaphragm valve, which has two variations. The first variation is the duck-bill or fish-mouth valve. When the bag is compressed, the gas leaving the bag expands the diaphragm valve, occluding the exhalation ports and opening the duck-bill portion, which directs gas flow to the patient's airways (Figure 5.17). When the bag is released, the diaphragm valve returns to its normal configuration, allowing the patient to exhale out the exhalation ports. The bag then refills through the bag inlet one-way valve. Examples of this type of manual resuscitator are the Laerdal, Hudson Lifesaver II, and the disposable Pulmanex from LDS.

The second variation of the diaphragm-type valve is the diaphragm/leaf valve. When the bag is compressed, the diaphragm is pushed to the left, occluding the exhalation ports and the leaf valve opens directing gas to the patient (Figure 5.18). Once the bag is released, the diaphragm returns to its normal position, the patient exhales through the exhalation ports, and the bag is refilled from the bag inlet one-way valve. Examples of this type of resuscitator are the Bennett

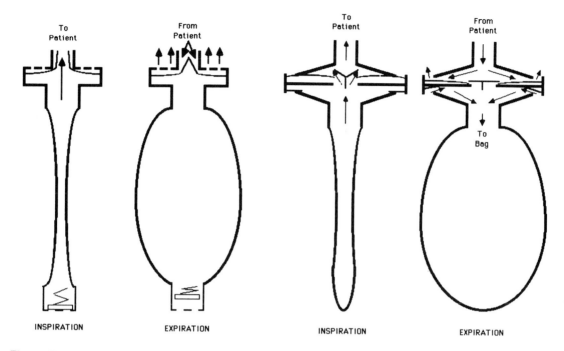

Figure 5.17 Duck-bill / Fush-mouth resuscitator valve.

Figure 5.18 Diaphragm / Leaf resuscitator valve.

PMR, the High Oxygen PMR, the PMR II, the AIRbird, the Hudson Lifesaver and Robertshaw manual self-inflating resuscitators. The AMBU E-2 also falls into this category but does not have an outer diaphragm and uses the one-way valve to occlude the exhalation port on inspiration (Figure 5.19).

Resuscitators bags come with an outlet of 15 mm inside diameter (ID) and 22 mm outside diameter (OD.) The 15 mm ID will fit onto an endotracheal or tracheostomy tube while the 22 mm OD will fit into a standard face mask. Manual resuscitators have been shown to be able to deliver 40–60% oxygen, dependent upon the flow of oxygen added to the bag, bag compression volume, and bag re-expansion time.[4] In order to achieve high oxygen percentages, such as 100%, a reservoir and adequate oxygen flow are required.

Gas Powered Resuscitators

Gas-powered resuscitators are pressure-limited, demand valve units (Figure 5.20). The pressure to be delivered to the patient is controlled by a diaphragm and spring as described earlier for reducing valves. Inspiration is initiated by activating a switching or cycling mechanism, which allows gas to flow from the demand valve to the patient. Once the pressure in the resuscitator reaches the level of the spring tension, the poppet valve closes and flow into the unit stops. A switching mechanism closes and exhalation occurs. Some units allow the patient to "assist" and will cycle into inspiration in response to negative pressure generated by the patient. Examples of this type of resuscitator are the Hudson Elder Valve and Robertshaw Demand Valve.

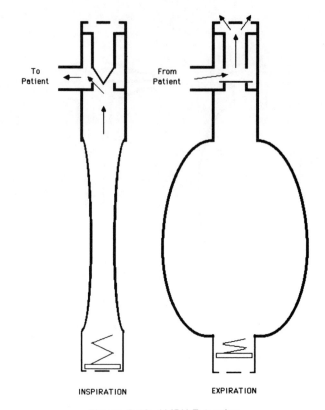

INSPIRATION   EXPIRATION

Figure 5.19 AMBU E-2 valve.

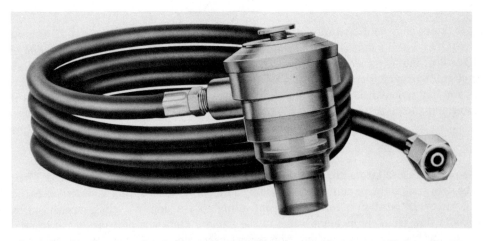

Figure 5.20 Gas powered resuscitator, demand valve unit. Courtesy of Hudson Oxygen Therapy, Tehelcula, CA.

The advantages of gas-powered resuscitators are that they supply 100% oxygen and are easily used by individuals with varying amounts of training. The major disadvantage is that being pressure-limited, there is no good way of estimating delivered volumes. In addition, the respiratory care practitioner cannot get the same indications as to changes in airways resistance or lung compliance as with a manual resuscitator.

References

1. Shapiro B. A., Harrison R. A., and Trout C. A. Clinical application of respiratory Care. 2nd ed. Chicago: Year Book Medical Publishers, Inc., 1979.
2. Dorsch J. A. and Dorsch S. E. Understanding anesthesia equipment: Construction, care, and complications. Baltimore: The Williams & Wilkins Co., 1975.
3. Caldwell S. L. and Sullivan K. N. Artificial airways. In Burton G. G. and Hodgkin J. E., editors: Respiratory care: A guide to clinical practice. 2nd ed. Philadelphia: J.B. Lippincott Co., 1984.
4. McPherson S. P. Respiratory therapy equipment. 3rd ed. St Louis: The CV Mosby Co., 1985.
5. Greenbaum J. M., et al. Esophageal obstruction during oxygen administration. Chest 1974; 65:188.
6. Carroll R. G. Evaluation of tracheal tube cuff designs. Crit Care Med 1973; 1:45.
7. Cunliffe AC, et al. Hazards from plastics sterilized by ethylene oxide. Br Med J 1967; 2:575.
8. Selecky P. A. Tracheostomy: A review of present-day indications, complications, and care. Heart Lung 1974; 3:272.
9. Baier H., et al. Effect of airway diameter, suction catheters and the bronchofiberscope on airflow in endotracheal and tracheostomy tubes Heart Lung 1976; 5:235.

ACKNOWLEDGMENTS AND REFERENCES

References

6 *Pressure-Limited Respirators*

Pressure-limited respirators or ventilators are most frequently used in home care to augment the patient's own breaths. They are particularly useful when the patient is unable to take slow, deep breaths during the course of an aerosol treatment.

Intermittent Positive Pressure Breathing (IPPB) was first described by Motley and Cournard and the first IPPB machine was introduced by V. Ray Bennett in 1945. Pressure-limited ventilators have also been used to support patients with compromised ability to breath on their own, but generally, this is restricted to short-term use and volume-limited ventilators are preferred for longer term support. Pressure-limited respirators can be used as a back-up ventilator however. The most common side effect in intermittent positive pressure breathing is by far hyperventilation and its accompanied side effects. These are most frequently noted clinically as lightheadedness and tingling of the extremities. It is also important to remember that elevated oxygen levels should not be used on patients with a hypoxic respiratory drive. A complete description of indications and precautions associated with IPPB are found elsewhere.[1,2]

Manually-Cycled, Pressure-Limited Respirators

Simple, venturi-powered, intermittent positive pressure devices that are manually controlled, can be driven from a cylinder of compressed gas or a pneumatic compressor. A tee or wye allows source gas to vent during the expiratory phase. When the patient wants to start inspiration, the thumb port on the tee or wye is occluded causing the pressurized source gas to be directed to (1) the jet of the venturi and (2) the jet of the nebulizer (Figure 6.1). The source gas that flows

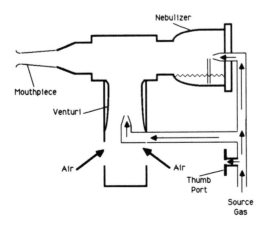

Figure 6.1 Manually-cycled, pressure-limited respirator.

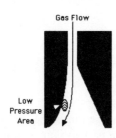

Gas Flow

Low
Pressure
Area

Figure 6.2 Coanda effect.

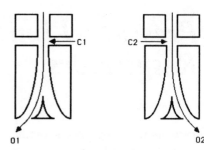

C1

C2

01

02

Figure 6.3 A flip-flop fluidic element.

to the jet nebulizer is responsible for creating aerosol while the gas supplying the venturi jet builds the positive pressure into the circuit through the venturi tube. When the patient has received a positive pressure breath, the thumb port is released and exhalation occurs. Since the thumb port is the cycling mechanism, the patient can be instructed to hold the thumb part closed and hold his breath at the end of inspiration which will provide a breath hold that is helpful in improving the distribution of the inhaled aerosols within the lungs.[3]

Examples of manually cycled pressure limited respirators are the Ohio Hand-E-Vent and the Bird Asthmastik.

Fluidic-Cycled, Pressure-Limited Respirators

Another type of simple pressure-limited device for intermittent positive pressure is the fluidic-controlled unit. This unit uses the Coanda effect to cause a gas stream to adhere to a wall. A pocket of turbulence makes the gas stream form an air foil over this area of turbulence (Figure 6.2). The air foil causes the gas molecules to travel faster, reducing the lateral pressure of the gas, similar to Bernoulli's effect. This decreased pressure area is what causes the gas stream to adhere to the wall.

These simple fluidic respirators utilize a fluidic element called the flip-flop. The source gas enters and the gas stream adheres to one out-flow tract, in this case, O_1 (Figure 6.3). The gas flow will adhere to the wall and remain in the O_1 out-flow position until a sufficient positive pressure force is generated at C_2 and it will then flip to out-flow tract O_2. In order to flip the flow from O_2 back to O_1, a positive pressure force can be exerted at C_1 or a negative pressure can be exerted at C_2, which can be a patient's inspiratory effort (this is the case when this principle is employed in an intermittent positive pressure breathing device.)

Figure 6.4 shows an example of using a flip-flop fluidic component in an IPPB device. The gas stream adheres to the wall of the right hand flow tract, which directs flow to the patient on inspiration. Once sufficient pressure has built up during the inspiratory phase, the pressure is transmitted back to C_1 forcing the flow to the other tract, thus allowing expiration to occur. When the patient is ready to initiate another inspiration, he must only generate enough negative pressure to

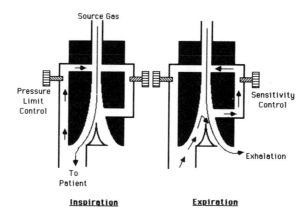

Source Gas

Pressure
Limit
Control

Sensitivity
Control

Exhalation

To
Patient

Inspiration   **Expiration**

Figure 6.4 Flip-flop incorporated into an IPPB device.

draw the flow back to the inspiratory tract, where it will remain until enough pressure builds up to switch the flow back to the expiratory side. Two small needle valves serve as pressure limit and sensitivity adjustments. The more the needle valves are opened, the more pressure from the gas stream enters the respective control port, and the less pressure needed to switch the flow to the other tract, i.e., a lower pressure limit during inspiration and less negative pressure required on the part of the patient to initiate inspiration.

Examples of units which employ this principle are units produced by Mine Safety Appliances and the Retec by Cavitron.

Bennett Therapy Units

The first Bennett IPPB machine was produced in 1945 by V. Ray Bennett. Two basic models were produced subsequent to the initial models, the TV-2P and the PV-3P, and they were widely used in the home and in hospitals.[3] The only difference was that the TV-2P was designed to be mounted on a large cylinder of compressed gas, and the PV-3P was mounted on a pedestal with a hose to be connected piped-in gases (Figures 6.5A and 6.5B). In both instances the powering gas pressure should be about 50 psig.

The diluter regulator is the mechanism that provides the flow characteristics of the Bennett Therapy Units. The diluter regulator is an adjustable reducing valve that acts as a demand valve to supply gas to the circuit to achieve the pre-set pressure (Figure 6.5C). The principle design of the diluter regulator is that of a simple reducing valve with a diaphragm that equilibrates spring tension and gas pressure. The black knob on the face of the Bennett units adjusts the spring tension, and therefore the gas pressure limit. As gas pressure drops, the spring pushes the diaphragm opening the poppet valve. This allows source gas to enter the diluter regulator until the gas pressure equals the spring tension. Once the gas pressure in the diluter regulator equals the venturi's pressure, the one-way flap on the entrainment port closes and the jet flow supplies the gas flow

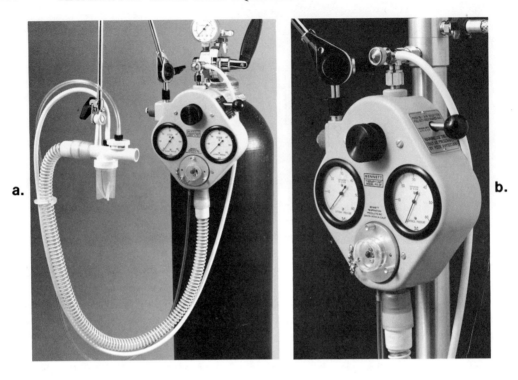

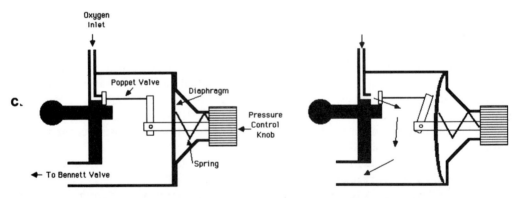

Figure 6.5 A–B Bennett TV-2PP, PV-30 models. **C** Bennett diluter regulator.

into the diluter regulator. When the two forces are equal the diaphragm returns to the upright position and the poppet valve closes, stopping gas flow into the diluter regulator. The diluter regulator acts as a demand valve, with the flowrate of gas being dependent upon the pressure gradient between the diluter regulator and the patient circuit. This normally provides a decelerating flow pattern (Figure 6.6). The Bennett units can deliver peak pressures from 1–35 cm H_2O pressure.

Gas from the diluter regulator enters the top of the Bennett valve (Figure 6.7). During exhalation, the Bennett valve is closed and the valve drum blocks flow from the diluter regulator from

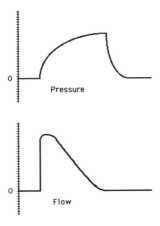

Figure 6.6 Flow and pressure patterns in the Bennett Therapy units.

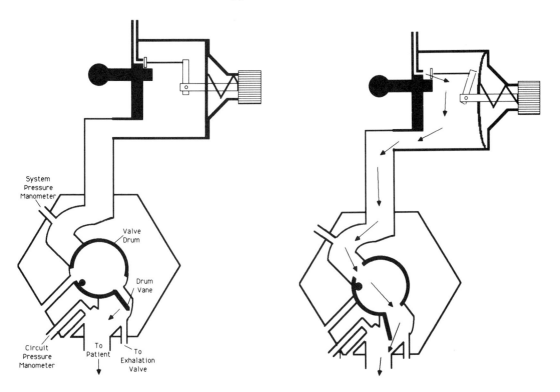

Figure 6.7 Bennett valve operation.

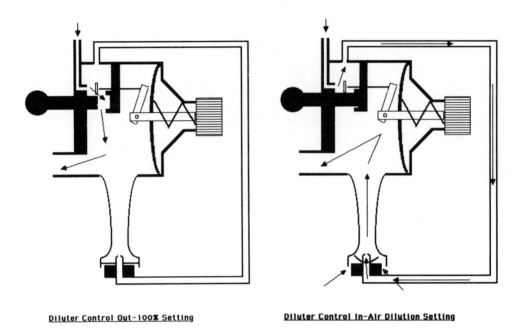

Diluter Control Out-100% Setting   **Diluter Control In-Air Dilution Setting**

Figure 6.8 Air dilution and 100% settings in the Bennett unit.

passing through the Bennett valve. When the patient starts to take a breath, the negative pressure in the patient circuit causes the drum vane to move to the right, opening the Bennett valve. Once the Bennett valve is open, gas from the diluter regulator can flow through to the patient circuit and to the exhalation valve through the exhalation valve port. As flow from the diluter regulator drops during inspiration due to the decreasing pressure gradient between the diluter regulator and the patient circuit, the Bennett valve gradually starts to close due to the counter weight. Finally when the flow through Bennett valve reaches 1–3 L/min, the force of the flow against the drum vane is not sufficient to keep the the valve open and the counter weigh causes the valve to swing shut and exhalation occurs. The dump port allows the gas within the Bennett valve and the exhalation valve and line to vent to atmosphere during exhalation. Another port provides a bleed so that the valve does not flutter when the initial high flow of gas passes through the Bennett valve. Two other ports supply the two pressure manometers. The port above the Bennett valve supplies the control pressure manometer and the port below the valve supplies the system (patient circuit) pressure manometer.

The diluter regulator has a control that allows the selection of air dilution or 100% source gas. When the control is in the out position, source gas passes directly into the diluter regulator and on to the patient circuit (Figure 6.8). If the control is pushed inward, source gas is directed to the jet of a venturi which entrains room air. The flow characteristics are the same for both settings since the diluter regulator functions as a demand valve on both settings (Figure 6.6).

The oxygen percentage range delivered when the machine is supplied with oxygen as a source gas can vary anywhere from 40–100%, depending upon patient/system resistance and compliance. The average is in the 60–65% oxygen range, but can vary widely from patient to patient, so an oxygen analyzer should be used to assure delivery of required oxygen percentage.

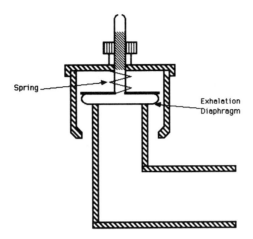

Figure 6.9 Bennett expiratory retard.

When compressed air is used as a source gas, the Bennett unit should be set on air dilution so that room air is entrained and the air source gas is conserved.

Accurate oxygen percentages can be achieved by powering the unit with gas from an oxygen blender which mixes oxygen and air, and setting the unit air diluter to the 100% setting.

Low oxygen percentages can also be obtained by using compressed air as the power source gas and attaching an oxygen accumulator (supplied by Bennett) to the air entrainment port.

The nebulizer control in the Bennett units is a simple needle valve that adjusts the continuous flow of source gas to the jet of the nebulizer. If the Bennett is being supplied with oxygen as a source gas, increasing nebulizer flows will increase the percentage of oxygen delivered to the patient.

The Bennett breathing circuit offers the option of an expiratory retard attachment to reduce the opening through which expiration occurs. As the nut in the attachment is loosened, a spring pushes the exhalation diaphragm downward closer to the shoulder of the exhalation valve (Figure 6.9). Application of this procedure has been suggested as beneficial in reducing air trapping in patients with chronic obstructive pulmonary disease.[1] Caution must be used not to occlude the expiratory flow tract too much or the patient may initiate another inspiration before exhalation is complete, actually causing or increasing air trapping. In addition, expiratory retard does increase mean airway pressure and may contribute to decreasing cardiac output.

The Bennett AP Compressor Units

Another type of IPPB device is the Bennett AP unit. Both versions have an electrically powered compressor built in to supply the source gas. The main flow of compressed air flows to the jet of a venturi which entrains additional air (Figure 6.10). In place of the diluter regulator there is a simple spring-disc pop-off which limits peak inspiratory pressure. As the spring tension is increased against the disc, the higher the gas pressure necessary to force the disc from its seat, allowing the gas to vent to atmosphere. Once the pop-off is opened, the gas vents out of the pressure

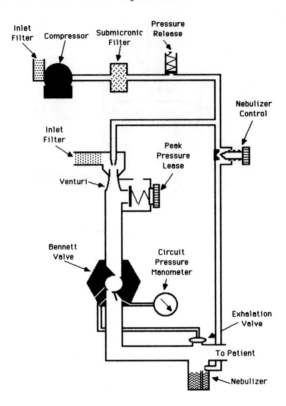

Figure 6.10 Bennett AP series schematic.

control, flow through the Bennett valve stops, and the valve closes allowing expiration to occur. When the patient opens the Bennett valve as he starts another inspiration, the spring-disc reseats as the supply gas flows to the patient, until pressure builds up sufficiently to unseat the spring-disc.

Another line from the compressor supplies compressed air to the nebulizer control (Figure 6.10). The nebulizer control is a simple needle valve, as found in the Bennett TV and PV units, which provides an adjustable continuous flow of gas to the nebulizer. If oxygen percentages above room air are necessary, the nebulizer line can be connected to a 100% oxygen source and thus allowing for the inspired air to be elevated above 21%.

There are two types of these units, the Bennett AP-4 and the AP-5. They are essentially the same machine except that the AP-4 has a support arm and a fold-down cover on the face of the case. The pressure and flow characteristics of the AP units are the same as for the Therapy units. The Bennett AP series, however, delivers slightly lower peak pressures (1–30 cm H_2O pressure) than the Therapy units.

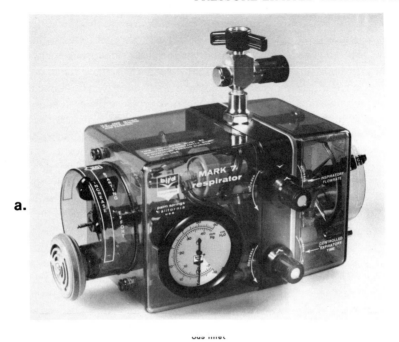

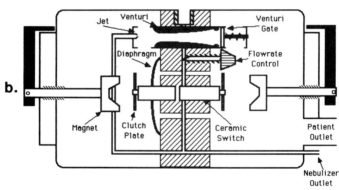

Figure 6.11 A Bird Mark 7. Courtesy of Bird Products Corp., Palm Springs, CA. **B** Bird Mark 7 Schematic.

Bird Mark Series

The Bird Mark 7 (Figure 6.11A), introduced in 1957 by Forrest Bird, was the principal design for all of Bird's IPPB units. Subsequent models provided additional capabilities or modified function, but retained the Mark 7's basic principle of operation.

The Bird Mark 7 uses magnetic attraction as an opposing force in controlling gas pressure. The Bird is separated into two halves by a diaphragm that is connected to a ceramic switch (Figure 6.11B). One side is always open to atmospheric pressure and the other to patient circuit pressure. Two magnets and metal clutch plates provide adjustments for the pressure required to move the diaphragm and ceramic switch from side to side. To start inspiration, the patient must generate enough negative pressure through the circuit to pull the diaphragm to the right. The adjustment of the proximity of the magnet to the clutch plate on the other side (atmospheric side) determines the amount of negative pressure that the patient must generate to move the diaphragm and switch to the right. Adjustment of this magnet provides sensitivity control. The closer the clutch plate is to the magnet on the atmospheric side, the more negative pressure the patient must create to force the diaphragm and switch to the right. Once the diaphragm and switch are moved to the right, source gas can flow through the flow control and on through the ceramic switch. The main flow of source gas travels to the jet of a venturi, entraining room air and providing the bulk of gas flow to the patient during inspiration. Another flow of gas travels to the nebulizer and exhalation valve. The flow of gas to the jet of the venturi and the nebulizer jet is determined by the flowrate control on the front of the unit. This control is a simple needle valve that regulates the flow of gas through it, depending on the size of its adjustable orifice. During inspiration, the venturi initially supplies the major flow of gas into the patient circuit. As pressure in the breathing circuit nears the pressure in the venturi, the venturi valve gate closes and gas flows instead into the atmospheric pressure side of the Bird. The gas flow into the patient circuit throughout the remainder of inspiration is supplied by the nebulizer. When oxygen is used as the source gas, the Bird Mark 7 delivers higher average oxygen percentage (70–85%) than the Bennett Therapy units. Again the percentage may vary widely from patient to patient so the actual percentage should be checked with an on oxygen analyzer. The reasons that the Bird delivers higher oxygen percentage can be explained mechanically.

The venturi gate has a spring tension of 2 cm H_2O pressure, so the venturi's peak pressure is never reached in the breathing circuit side of the Bird. Once the venturi gate closes, the remainder of gas to the patient is 100% oxygen from the nebulizer.

Also, once the venturi gate closes, the oxygen passing through the jet of the venturi accumulates in the atmospheric pressure side of the unit to be entrained by the venturi when the next inspiration is initiated.

Another important consideration related to the venturi gate is that if the sensitivity magnet were set to require more than a -2 cm H_2O pressure to initiate inspiration, the patient can open the venturi gate instead of triggering inspiration.

Once the pressure in the patient circuit side of the Bird is sufficient to overcome the attraction of the magnet to the clutch plate on that side, the diaphragm is pushed to the other side and the switch stops flow to the jet of the venturi, the nebulizer, and the exhalation valve. The exhalation valve opens and exhalation occurs.

The Bird Mark 7 is also equipped with an air mix control that can be pushed in to provide 100% concentration of source gas. When the control is pushed in, the gas from the flowrate control bypasses the venturi and is directed out a small port, past a flap, and directly into the breathing circuit side of the Bird. Since there is no entrainment of gas and the breathing circuit side is being supplied directly from high pressure source gas, the flow pattern is changed to a constant, or square wave (Figure 6.12).

The expiratory timer mechanism of the Bird Mark 7 provides the ability to time cycle the Bird into inspiration. During inspiration, the timer cartridge is charged with gas and the arm moves to the left. When inspiration ends, the flow of source gas into the cartridge stops. If the needle valve expiratory time control is closed, there is no exit for gas from the cartridge and it remains

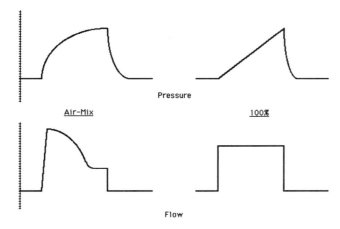

Pressure

Air-Mix   100%

Flow

Figure 6.12 Flow and pressure patterns in the Bird Mark 7.

charged and nonfunctional. When the needle valve is opened, gas exits from the cartridge during exhalation thus allowing the spring to push the arm to the right; the arm then hits the clutch metal plate and ceramic switch, triggering the Mark 7 into inspiration. When inspiration begins, the cartridge is recharged and ready for the next expiration. The wider the needle valve is opened, the quicker gas will leak past it, and the sooner the gas will leave the cartridge allowing the arm to start inhalation. Therefore, the more the needle valve is opened, the shorter exhalation time will be. The expiratory timer is normally not used during the administration of IPPB, but can be used to establish a machine ventilatory rate if the Mark 7 is used for short term ventilatory support.

The Bird circuit has an optional retard cap to slow expiratory flow by altering the port size through which expiration can occur (Figure 6.13). Again, caution must be exercised to be certain that exhalation is not prolonged so much that exhalation is not complete. Expiratory retard does increase mean airway pressure and can contribute to decreased cardiac output.

The Bird Mark 10 is essentially the Mark 7 with a flow accelerator to overcome leaks and does not have an air mix control; the Mark 10 is always set for air mix.

The Bird Mark 8 is the same as the Mark 7 but also has an additional flow of gas designed for negative expiratory pressure. This flow of gas occurs during the expiratory cycle of respiration and it powers a venturi in the exhalation manifold that entrains the patient's expired gas. Negative expiratory pressure was intended to decrease mean airway pressure and its effect on venous return and cardiac output. However, negative expiratory pressure tends to promote air trapping, especially in patients with chronic lung disease. The expiratory flow from the Mark 8 can also be used to power the Bird pneumobelt which is placed around the patients upper abdomen. Then with the expiratory retard in place, the pneumobelt helps compress the abdomen similar to abdominal breathing.

The Bird Mark 9 has larger magnets than the other models that allows for pressures up to 200 mm Hg. This unit also utilizes a second venturi jet to provide higher inspiratory flow rates. The Mark 9 also has expiratory flow capabilities similar to the ones in the Mark 8.

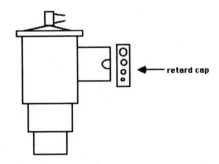

Figure 6.13 Bird exhalation valve and expiratory retard.

The Bird Mark 14 combines the higher capabilities of the Bird Mark 9 plus the flow accelerator capabilities of the Mark 10. The Mark 14 does not have expiratory flow capabilities.

A second generation of Bird Respirators include the Mark 7A and 8A. These units use the basic design of their respective predecessor and have an apneustic (pressure) plateau capability. The apneustic plateau is accomplished by providing the capabilities for a constant flow of gas (from the nebulizer) to enter the patient circuit for an adjustable period of time with the exhalation valve remaining closed after the end of delivery of gas to the patient circuit from the venturi. This provides a type of "breath hold" that has been reported to be advantageous for aerosol deposition and distribution.[4,5] After the timed period is ended, the flow stops and exhalation occurs. Other changes in the Mark 7A and 8A are:

- The Air-Mix control was eliminated and both units always entrain air.
- A flow accelerator has been added.
- An external filter can be added to the left (ambient) side of the Bird and can be attached directly to the venturi entrainment port. Oxygen can be added to provide increased delivered oxygen levels.
- The flowrate control adjusts only the flow of gas to the the venturi and the nebulizer flow is always constant.
- The expiratory timer is capable of starting inspiration with PEEP pressures up to 35 cm H_2O pressure.
- Higher pressure limit capabilities are available and there is a port in the right (high pressure) side to accommodate a pressure relief and safety inlet valve.

A complete description of these and other Bird models can be found elsewhere.[3]

Other Bird Models

The Bird Mark 1 was designed to simplify the principles of operation of the standard Bird models in order to make the unit more simple and more compact. The magnet/clutch plate arrangement was reversed and the Mark 1 (Figure 6.14) has only one magnet in the center and two clutch plates on either side (Figure 6.13). Sensitivity and pressure limit settings are made by internally adjusting the location of the clutch plates in relation to the magnet. A separate chamber

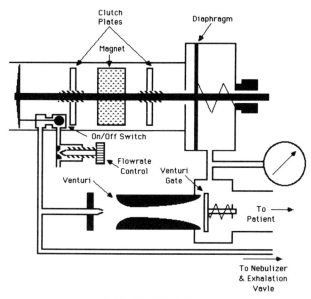

Figure 6.14 Bird Mark I schematic.

contains a diaphragm that communicates with the patient circuit. As the patient withdraws gas from the patient circuit, the diaphragm moves to the right and opens the flow of gas from the needle valve flowrate control to the venturi, nebulizer, and exhalation valve. As pressure builds up in the patient circuit, the diaphragm moves back to the left until the right clutch plate is moved away from the magnet. This stops flow into the Bird and exhalation occurs.

The flow characteristics of the Bird Mark 1 are similar to those for the air-mix setting of other Bird models. The peak pressure range for the Mark 1 is 1–25 cm H_2O pressure.

In 1973 the Bird Mark 1 sequencing servo was introduced. This unit provided independent, external controls for pressure and sensitivity. The pressure limit was increased to 60 cm H_2O pressure with a 100 cm H_2O pressure limit option available.

The Minibird is essentially a Mark 1 placed into a case. A manometer displays the circuit pressure and one knob on the front adjusts flowrate. Pressure and sensitivity adjustments are made by adjusting the location of the clutch plates internally.

The Minibird II contains the Mark 1 sequencing servo plus apneustic plateau capabilities. The Minibird II has external adjustments for flow, pressure, sensitivity, and apneustic flow time. The pressure limit range is from 0–60 cm H_2O pressure.

The Portabird incorporates the Mark 1 with an internal compressor to provide source gas. The one external knob adjusts the flowrate, while sensitivity and pressure adjustments are internal. Performance capabilities are the same as for the Mark 1.

The Portabird III uses an internal compressor and the Mark 1 sequencing servo so that adjustments can be externally made for flow, pressure, and sensitivity. The pressure range is increased to 0–60 cm H_2O pressure.

A complete description of these units can be found elsewhere.[3]

The nebulizer, manifold, and mouth piece of the circuit should be rinsed and dried after each treatment. A disposable circuit should be considered expendable, discarded periodically, and not be decontaminated for reuse. A permanent circuit should be cleaned with a mild soap or chemical decontamination agent suitable for use with IPPB circuits at least weekly or according to manufacturers recommendations. Disposables should be discarded according to the manufacturer's or supplier's directions.

Cuirass Ventilators

The use of negative pressure ventilators started with the iron lung. The first iron lung was designed by Drinker and Shaw in 1928, was first produced by the J.H. Emerson Co., and is still in production today. Negative pressure is supplied to the patient's entire body from the neck down during inspiration. Iron lungs have been produced in infant and children sizes also. Iron lungs are not as frequently used in home care today as the cuirass or chest shell is because of inaccessibility of the patient, tank shock, abdominal pooling of blood, the space required for the equipment, and the ease of use of the chest piece. The difficulty of ventilating patients with airway disorders or pulmonary disease can be a significant problem with both units. However, the cuirass, a rigid shell negative pressure ventilator, has been improved over earlier models and is more capable of ventilating patients than units of the past. Negative pressure ventilators find application in patients with neuromuscular disease and patients with pulmonary disease who require periodic or night time ventilatory support.[6] Negative pressure ventilation is not indicated for patients with sleep apnea secondary to upper airway obstruction.[6]

If negative pressure is used for short-term or nocturnal support, there may be no need for back-up ventilation capabilities and only provision for supplemental oxygen may be required. However, if the patient requires negative pressure ventilation on a continuous basis, or the majority of the time, back-up ventilation is advisable.[6] This can be in the form of a manual resuscitator or a pressure-limited respirator. Patients should be instructed not to eat or drink while being ventilated with negative pressure because the possibility of aspiration is high. Patients may complain of chills while on negative pressure as a result of air drafts over the body from leaks around the enclosure. This is especially true of patients using the poncho-type of cuirass and can be corrected by the patient wearing sufficient night time apparel.[6]

The original cuirass was a rigid shell designed by Drinker and Collins in 1939 in hopes of reducing abdominal pooling of blood (tank shock.) The rigid shell is still available from Lifecare in a variety of sizes (Figure 6.15). They can also be made from a cast of the patient's chest, but this customizing can be expensive.[6] The rigid shell can be worn in the sitting position also, so that patients requiring continuous ventilatory support can wear the chest piece while sitting up in a chair or wheel chair.

The poncho type of chest piece is available from J.H. Emerson. The poncho encloses the patient from the neck to the hips and covers a quonset shaped grid that is placed over the patient's chest (Figures 6.16A & B). The grid provides the gas volume around the chest so that the applied negative pressure can work. The patient can get in and out of the poncho fairly easily and the device does not have to be custom fitted to the individual patient.[6] The poncho wrap is available in infant, child, medium adult, and large adult sizes. However, leaks can be a problem around the

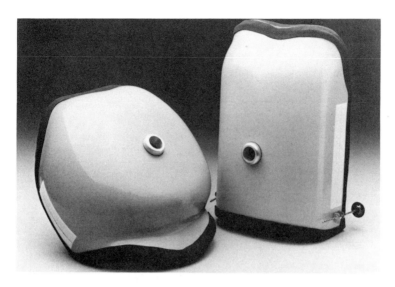

Figure 6.15 Rigid shell cuirass chest pieces. Courtesy of Lifecare, Lafayette, CO.

neck, arms, and especially the hips. A better seal is possible with the total body suit produced by New Tech Associates, which is custom made for the patient but considerably more expensive.[6] A sleeping bag unit is also available.

The negative pressure applied by these devices is produced with a vacuum-type blower that acts as a controller. J.H. Emerson's original model was powered by a brushed motor but later models used a brushless motor. Three controls provide for adjustment of maximum negative pressure, inspiratory time, and expiratory time and can provide rates up to 30–40 breaths/minute and negative pressures of −60 cm H_2O pressure.[6] A modification of this unit uses a cannula to sense inspiratory effort. A negative inspiratory effort of 0.5–1.0 cm H^2O pressure is needed to trigger an assist breath and exhalation is triggered when no inspiratory effort is detected. The unit acts purely as an assistor with no back-up rate capabilities. Since the patient sets the rate and I:E (inspiration to expiration) ratios, the controls for inspiratory and expiratory time have been eliminated on this version.

The Lifecare 170-C (Figure 6.16B) and PVV negative pressure ventilators come in two versions. The AC current model is capable of generating negative pressures to −80 cm H2O while the AC/DC model can generate pressures to −60 cm H_2O.

Care of the cuirass is fairly straightforward. The chest piece should be wiped clean daily with a mild soap and disinfected according to the manufacturer's guidelines. The negative pressure generator should be on a preventative maintenance program as outlined by the manufacturer.

The Puritan-Bennett Thompson Maxivent (Figure 6.17A) is a rotary compressor driven unit that can be used to deliver positive pressure up to 80 cm H_2O, or to generate negative pressures to −70 cm H_2O, or both. The positive pressure can be used in the traditional positive pressure mode to the upper airway or can power a pneumobelt (Figure 6.17B). The negative pressure can be used to power a cuirass ventilator. The rate is variable from 8–24 with a fixed 1:2 I:E ratio, and with flowrates up to 150 L/min.

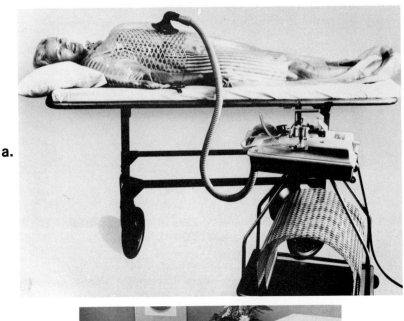

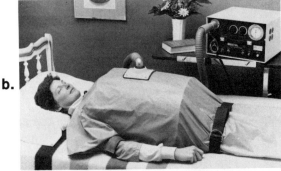

Figure 6.16 A Poncho and grid cuirass. **B** Monagram 170C Negative Pressure Respirator. Rebuilt by Lifecare with Poncho and Grid Cuirass.

The Maxivent is designed to be powered by 110 volt household electricity. A low-pressure alarm sounds in the event that at least 10 cm H_2O pressure is generated for 12 seconds in either the positive or negative phase of operation. The alarm will also sound if the machine fails to cycle within 12 seconds or should there be a power failure for 12 seconds or more. The alarm is deactivated by either a positive or negative pressure of 12 cm H_2O pressure. A patient call switch can also be connected.

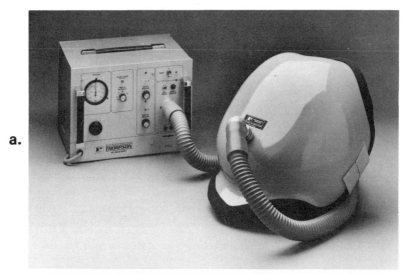

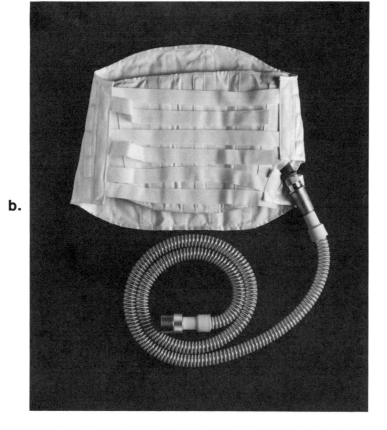

Figure 6.17 A Puritan Bennett Thompson Maxivent. Our grateful thanks to Puritan-Bennett's Portable Ventilator Division, Boulder, Colorado, for their assistance in helping us develop this material. **B** Pneumobelt. Our grateful thanks to Puritan-Bennett's Portable Ventilator Division, Boulder, Colorado, for their assistance in helping us develop this material.

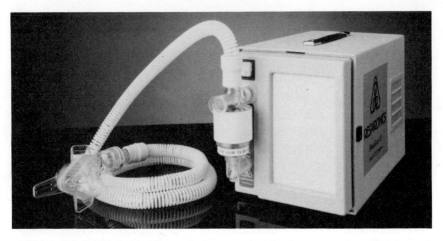

Figure 6.18 Respironic CPAP system. Courtesy of Respironics, Inc., Monroeville, PA.

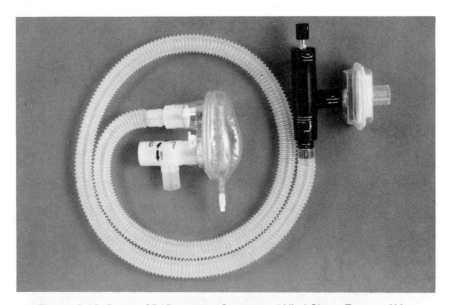

Figure 6.19 Downs CPAP system. Courtesy of Vital Signs, Totowa, NJ.

CPAP Devices

Continuous Positive Pressure Breathing (CPPB) was introduced in 1934 by Dr. Alvin Barach. The name was changed when this principle was used by Gregory for neonates in the 1970s to continuous positive airway pressure (CPAP). CPAP or CPPB has been shown to be effective in relieving sleep apnea related to upper airway obstruction.[6] Respironics produces the SleepEasy to provide Continuous Positive Airway Pressure for patients suffering from sleep apnea secondary to upper airway obstruction. The CPAP generator is a rotary blower and can be used for mask CPAP with the head gear supplied (Figure 6.18).

Vital Signs has the Downs venturi-powered pneumatic device available for generating CPAP. A needle valve controls the jet flow and, therefore, the total flow into the system (Figure 6.19).

Another needle valve adjusts the amount of additional oxygen that can be added to increase the percentage of oxygen delivered to the patient.

References

1. Spearman C. B., Shelton R. L., Egan D. F. Egan's Fundamentals of respiratory therapy. 4th ed. St Louis: The CV Mosby Co., 1982.
2. Ziment I. Intermittent positive pressure breathing. In G. G. Burton and J. E. Hodgkin, editors. Respiratory care: A guide to clinical practice. Philadelphia: J.P. Lippincott Co., 1977.
3. McPherson S. P. Respiratory therapy equipment. 3rd ed. St. Louis: The CV Mosby Co., 1985.
4. Miller W. F. Aerosol therapy in acute and chronic respiratory disease. Arch Intern Med 1973; 131:148.
5. Miller W. F. Fundamental principles of aerosol therapy Resp Care 1972; 17:295.
6. Paul W. L. and Downs J. B. Postoperative atelectasis: Intermittent positive pressure breathing, incentive spirometry, and face mask positive end-expiratory pressure. Arch Surg 1981; 116:861–863.

7 *Volume Limited Ventilators*

As discussed in Chapter 6, pressure-limited respirators can be used to provide ventilatory assistance for short periods of time, or most often as the initial method of supporting a patient's breathing. For long-term ventilatory life support in the home, volume-limited (cycled) ventilators are preferred primarily because changes in the patient's airways resistance and lung compliance will not alter the delivered tidal volumes as drastically as with a pressure-limited unit. In addition, volume-limited ventilators generally have more flexibility in regard to setting volumes, rates, PEEP, oxygen percentage, etc. and are usually equipped with more alarms as an alert to problems that might develop.

Many of the problems associated with mechanical ventilation have already been covered in previous chapters. The integrity of the circuit must be monitored to ensure that leaks do not reduce the delivered volume to the patient. The circuit should be changed every 24–48 hours and the humidifier should be refilled using aseptic technique so that microrganisms are not introduced. Controlling the inspired oxygen percentage is crucial, and this should be monitored frequently, or even continuously, to assure that it remains stable. The concentration of oxygen delivered by the ventilator should be checked any time a change in tidal volume or rate is made, because many volume ventilators designed for use in the home use a mixing chamber and the delivered oxygen may change with changes in minute volume.

The I:E ratio is important in ensuring that the patient has adequate opportunity to exhale so that air trapping does not occur. An I:E of 1:1.5 or 1:2 is a good starting point and will also keep mean airway pressure down. In some patients, especially those with flaccid airways, a longer expiratory time may be required. It should be noted that the longer the inspiratory portion of the ventilatory cycle, the higher the mean airway pressure will be and the greater the influence mechanical ventilation may have on reducing venous return and cardiac output. PEEP is employed to reduce intrapulmonary shunting and to improve arterial oxygen levels. A shunt fraction graph is often helpful in setting PEEP levels. PEEP does contribute to mean airway pressure so venous return and cardiac output may be decreased.

A complete description of mechanical ventilation and its side effects are found elsewhere.[1,2]

Piston Driven Volume Ventilators

The first volume ventilators were primarily piston driven ventilators. The first ventilator to be widely used in this country was the Emerson (Post-Op) 3-PV, first manufactured in 1964.[3] The Emerson 3-PV was also the first volume-limited piston ventilator to be used in ventilating patients in the home or in extended care facilities.

This type of piston-driven ventilator uses a rotary drive, which delivers a sine wave type flow pattern. As the drive wheel starts its forward rotation to deliver gas from the piston, the piston rod moves more vertically than horizontally, providing a slow movement of the piston (Figure 7.1).

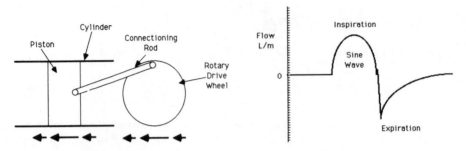

Figure 7.1 Rotary drive piston.

Figure 7.2 Sine wave flow pattern.

As the rod moves toward the top of the wheel, the motion of the rod is gradually more horizontal than vertical, which results in a higher forward speed of the piston, and a higher flow of gas from the piston cylinder. At the very top of the wheel's rotation, the motion of the rod and piston is nearly all in a horizontal fashion, with the fastest forward motion of the rod and piston and the highest flow from the piston cylinder. After the rod connection starts to move downward from the top of the drive wheel's rotation the horizontal movement gradually becomes more vertical as the rotation nears the bottom and the forward speed of the rod and piston decrease and the flow from the piston cylinder gradually drops. This mechanism provides the sine wave like flow pattern found in rotary drive piston ventilators (Figure 7.2).

Two reastats control the speed of the motor, which turns the drive wheel and moves the piston.[3] The return stroke speed is controlled by the reastat designated as expiratory time. The Emerson Post-Op, or 3-PV rotary drive piston draws gas from internal tubing type of reservoir on the return stroke of the piston (Figure 7.3).[3] This reservoir allows for the addition of oxygen to control the delivered oxygen percentage. The series of piping, or tubing, has a larger internal volume than the maximum stroke volume of the piston so that oxygen percentages can be calculated (see Chapter 2). Once the oxygen percentage is calculated, it should be monitored with an oxygen analyzer. The forward stroke of the piston is controlled by the inspiratory time control, another reastat that controls the speed of the motor during the inspiratory phase. The shorter the inspiratory time, the faster the motor speed. As the piston moves forward, gas is directed through a heated blow-by humidifier to the patient. Another smaller line sends gas to the exhalation valve to occlude it during the inspiratory phase. Once the forward stoke is completed, gas flow to the exhalation valve stops and the patient exhales past the exhalation valve. The expiratory time reastat controls the speed of the of the motor on the return stroke. The shorter the expiratory time the faster the motor speed during the return stroke. Together the inspiratory time and expiratory time set the control rate.

A assist option is available for the Emerson ventilator. It is a diaphragm that can sense negative pressure generated by the patient (Figure 7.4). When the patient attempts a breath, the diaphragm moves to the left in response to the reduced pressure, and depresses the microswitch. This causes maximum current to be sent to the motor during the remainder of the return stroke. The result is that the piston returns as quickly as possible to the starting point of inspiration. A delay of up to 600 msec. can result.[3]

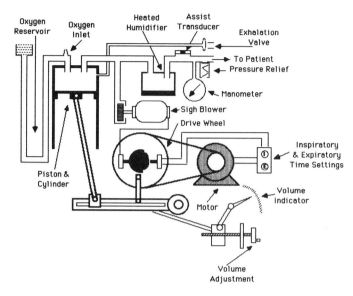

Figure 7.3 Emerson 3-PV ventilator schematic.

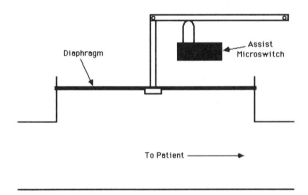

Figure 7.4 Emerson assist mechanism.

The humidification system on the Emerson is fashioned from a pressure cooker and functions as a blow-by type of heated humidifier.[3] Gas then flows through copper mesh.

An optional sigh blower is available that adds room air during the inspiratory phase.[3] The blower speed can be adjusted to deliver a pressure of up to 50–55 cm H_2O pressure and does reduce the F_IO_2 during sigh breaths unless modified.[3]

Life Products has several models of home care ventilators that are rotary drive piston driven. The original Life Products ventilator was the LP-3 (Figure 7.5) which was strictly a controller with a fixed 1:1 I:E ratio.[4] A brush type motor powers a rotary drive piston that produces a sine wave flow pattern.[4] Room air is drawn in past the intake check valve during the return stroke of the piston (Figure 7.6). On the forward stroke of the piston the intake valve is forced closed and

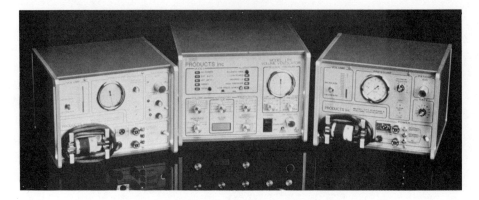

Figure 7.5 Life Products LP-3.

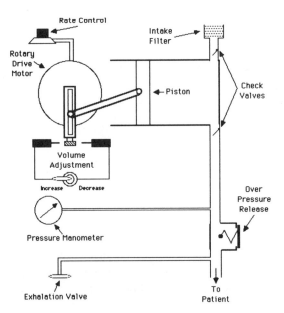

Figure 7.6 Life Products LP series schematic.

the gas from the cylinder is forced past the outlet check valve and on to the patient circuit. A small line supplies gas to the exhalation valve to occlude it during inspiration. Then during expiration, the exhalation diaphragm dumps allowing the patient circuit gas to vent into the room. The motor speed driving the piston determines the rate, which is adjustable from 8–30 breaths/minute.[5] Tidal volume is change by a rachet mechanism changing piston stroke volume. The rachet changes the piston stroke volume by 16ccs with each stroke of the piston, to reach the desired tidal volume setting.[4,5] The tidal volume range is from 0–3,000 ml.[5]

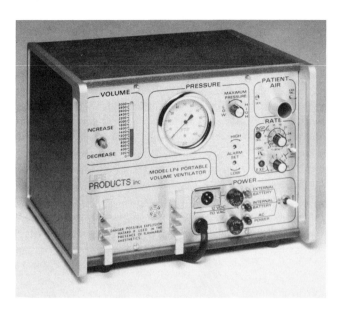

Figure 7.7 Life Products LP-4.

Oxygen percentage control is accomplished by bleeding oxygen into the inspiratory limb of the ventilator circuit. Changes in delivered minute volume will affect the delivered oxygen concentration and changes must be accompanied by analyzing the inspired gas.

The LP-3 has a rechargeable internal battery capable of powering the ventilator in case of power failure for up to 30–60 minutes.[5] The LP-3 can be powered by 12 volt internal or external DC current or 110 AC household current.

The LP-3 has high pressure and low pressure alarms. The low pressure alarm is activated if a contact mounted on a diaphragm does not engage an adjustable, fixed contact within a 10–15 second period, assuring that the set minimum pressure was reached. This same mechanism alarms if the set high pressure is exceeded and excessive pressure is vented.

The LP-4 (Figure 7.7) is basically an LP-3 with assist-control and IMV modes added. An assist sensor triggers inspiration if the patient draws the pressure in the circuit to below atmospheric pressure. In the IMV mode, the patient draws spontaneous breaths from either the IMV one-way valve added to the inspiratory limb of the circuit (Figure 7.8) or from the piston cylinder itself. If the optional IMV system is not used, the inspired oxygen concentration levels may fluctuate as the patient's minute volume changes.

During operation in assist-control or IMV, the upper rate control sets inspiratory time and a multiplier switch is used to differentiate between the assist-control and the IMV modes. The switch must be placed in the X1 position for assist-control operation and in the X10 postion for IMV.[4] The return stroke of the piston (maximum expiratory time) is controlled by the multiplier switch and the lower knob. The rate can be varied between 5–30 breaths/minute and tidal volume is adjustable from 0–3,000 ml as in the LP-3, except that each piston stroke changes the rachet so that the tidal volume is altered by 15 ml.[6] Peak pressures of up to 100 cm H_2O are possible with the LP-4.[6]

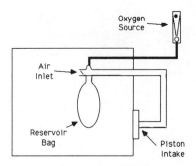

Figure 7.8 Optional IMV attachment for LP ventilators.

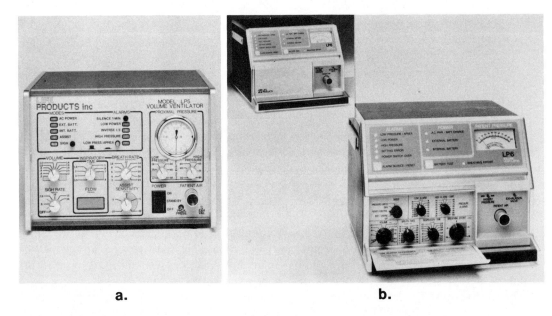

a.   b.

Figure 7.9 A Life Products LP-5 Ventilator. **B** Aequitron Medical Life Products LP-6.

The LP-4 can be operated by 12 volt internal or external DC current and both battery sources are self-charging to power the ventilator in the event of power failure. Low voltage, power failure, and apnea alarms in the IMV mode have been added along with low and high pressure alarms. The high and low pressure alarms are set with screwdriver adjustments on the front panel.

The LP-5 (Figure 7.9A) is based upon the same primary drive mechanism as its predecessors. The I:E ratio is variable in all modes of operation (control, assist-control, and IMV), but cannot be (inverse).[4] This is accomplished by having separate motor speeds for inspiration and expiration, controlled by the inspiratory time and rate controls. If the patient assists, maximum current is sent to the motor during the remainder of the return stroke, which is followed by a forward stroke providing inspiration. Control rate is adjustable from 2–28 breaths/minute and inspiratory time is adjustable from 0.6–3.5 seconds.[7] Tidal volume is adjustable from 100–2,200 ml, in 15 ml increments, with peak pressure capabilities of up to 80 cm H_2O pressure.[7]

During IMV with the low pressure/apnea button in the "out" position, operation the sensitivity is set at -10 cm H_2O pressure and the patient breathes through the piston and cylinder assembly. In this position, the low pressure alarm will activate when proximal pressure does not reach the low pressure setting. When the low pressure/apnea button is in the "in" position, the sensitivity is set to -1 or -2 cm H_2O pressure, and the assist light will illuminate but the ventilator will not cycle on spontaneous breaths. The apnea alarm will sound if no assist breaths occur sensed within 15 seconds.

Elevated inspired oxygen levels can be obtained by adding oxygen to the inspiratory limb of the patient circuit, as with the LP-3 and 4, or by attaching a reservoir to the piston cylinder intake. The sensitivity may be set as high as $+10$ cm H_2O pressure, making PEEP assist possible up to approximately that level.

The LP-5 has a sigh capability of delivering double the set tidal volume unless the pressure limit is reached. This is accomplished by the exhalation valve remaining inflated and the piston returns at maximum speed and the delivers another forward stroke. If less than double the tidal volume is desired for a sigh breath, the high pressure control can be set to limit the sigh volume and the sigh volume can be measured. Sighs can be activated by the manual sigh button or timed from 0–30 sighs per hour.[7]

The LP-5 has audible and visual alarms for low pressure, high pressure, apnea, low power, and inverse I:E ratio. The high presssure alarm cycles the ventilator into expiration. An alarm silence allows the alarms to be silenced for one minute. The inverse I:E alarm is triggered if the inspiratory time is set too low for the ventilator to deliver the tidal volume within one/half of the ventilatory cycle (I:E of 1:1).[7] As mentioned above, the low pressure/apnea alarm is user-switchable. In the "out" position, the unit will sound an alarm if the low pressure setting is not reached within a 15-second period. In the "in" position, the unit functions as an apnea alarm and will sound if no breathing effort is detected within 15 seconds.[7] The apnea alarm is automatically reset by a patient effort.[7] Mean inspiratory flowrate is digitally displayed. The LP-5 can be powered by three different power sources just as its predecessors.

The Life Products LP-6 (Figure 7.9B) is microprocessor controlled and is powered by a brushless motor.[4] The LP-6 can function in control (with the sensitivity set to lockout patient assist effort), assist-control, SIMV, and pressure-limited modes.[4] In the SIMV mode, the patient draws gas from the gas inlet, through a low resistance pathway in the pneumatic manifold. When the piston returns to the end of the return stroke and is ready for inspiration to begin, the next inspiratory effort from the patient initiates an SIMV, volume-delivered breath. During SIMV, the ventilator monitors the patient's inspiratory effort. If the patient fails to initiate a breath within 20 seconds, the apnea alarm sounds, and if the ventilator has an SIMV rate set of 1–5, the ventilator switches to a back-up ventilation mode and the ventilator will deliver 10 breaths per minute at the preset tidal volume.[8] If the SIMV rate is set at six breaths per minute or above, the ventilator will continue delivering the set SIMV rate.[8] The apnea alarm will not sound unless a mandatory breath fails to be delivered.[8] When set in the pressure-limit mode of operation, the high-pressure alarm/limit setting controls the pressure in the patient circuit during the inspiratory phase. The rate may be varied from 1–38 breaths per minute and the tidal volume is adjustable from 100–2,200 ml in 100 ml increments.[8] Inspiratory time is adjustable from 0.5–5.5 seconds.[8]

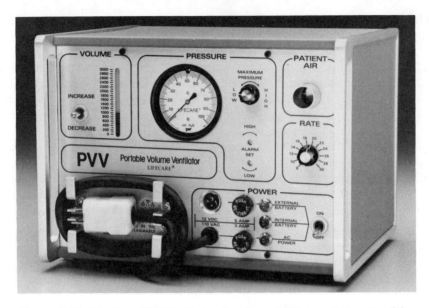

Figure 7.10 Life Care PVV Ventilator. Courtesy of Lifecare, Lafayette, CO.

The low-pressure alarm sounds if the set pressure is not reached on two consecutive breaths. The high-pressure/limit alarm can function as a pressure limit as described above, or, when set in the alarm position, the alarm sounds when the setting is exceeded and inspiration is ended. The LP-6 also has alarms for apnea, setting error, low power, and power switch over along with a 60-second audible alarm silence. The setting error alarm occurs if the settings made are outside the capabilities of the LP-6 (Inverse I:E).

Like its predecessors, the LP-6 can be powered by 12 volt or by household current. An internal battery can power the unit in the event of a power failure.

Optional accessories for the LP-6 include a remote alarm that is functional up to 200 feet from the ventilator and a printer that tracks alarm conditions and monitors ventilator performance.

Several volume-limited ventilators are produced by Lifecare. The PVV (Figures 7.10 and 7.11) is essentially the same as the Life Products LP-3 described above.

The PLV-100 (Figure 7.12) is a microprocessor controlled, linear drive piston volume ventilator that that is powered by a brushed motor and produces a square wave flow pattern.[4] Modes of operation include control, assist-control, and SIMV. During SIMV, the patient breathes spontaneous breaths from an H-type IMV system placed into the inspiratory limb of the patient circuit. The PLV-100 will allow a synchonized volume-limited breath five seconds before the next scheduled mandatory breath and will deliver the breath if the machine senses an inspiratory effort on the part of the patient.[9] If the patient does not initiate a breath during that five-second period, the PLV-100 delivers the mandatory breath at the timed interval. The unit then allows the patient to breathe from the H-type IMV system without triggering the SIMV breath until five seconds before the next mandatory breath is to be delivered. This five-second period can result in a fluctuation of the rate display which averages over a four breath sequence (Figure 7.13). The total (machine plus spontaneous) breaths per minute is displayed. Tidal volume range is 50–3,000 ml

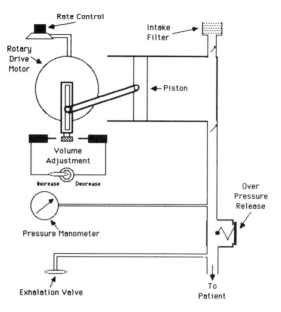

Figure 7.11 Lifecare PVV schematic.

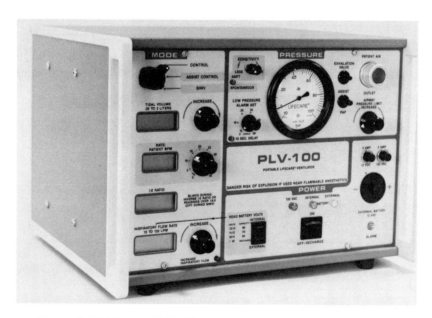

Figure 7.12 Lifecare PLV-100. Courtesy of Lifecare, Lafayette, CO.

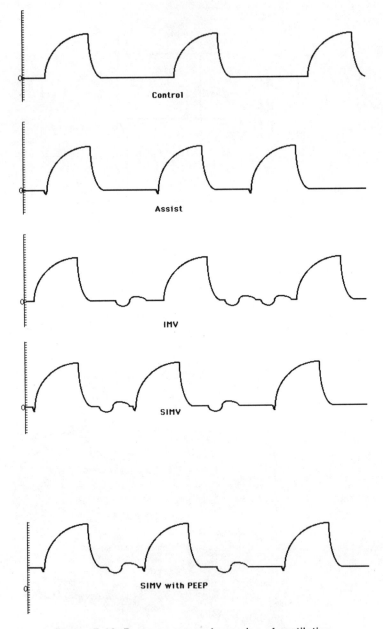

Figure 7.13 Pressure curves for modes of ventilation.

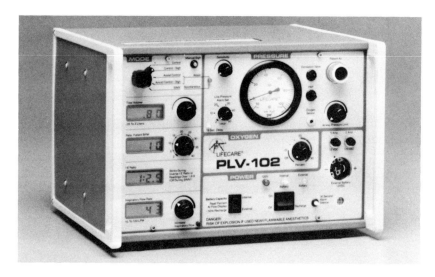

Figure 7.14 Lifecare PLV-102. Courtesy of Lifecare, Lafayette, CO.

and the set rate range is 2–40 breaths per minute. The PLV-100 has pressure delivery capabilities of up to 100 cm H_2O. Tidal volume, patient (total) rate, I:E ratio, and peak flowrate are digitally displayed on the front panel. The I:E display will blink with inverse I:E ratios of ratios over 1:9.9.[9] The rate display is an average of the preceeding 4 breaths. The PLV-100 is designed to increase the delivered flowrate if the inspiratory time is set too low to meet the other set parameters and if this occurs, a red LED will illuminate.[9] A rocker switch enables the operator to check the charge levels of the internal and external batteries. Sensitivity is adjustable from +3 to −6 cm H_2O pressure and is sensed through a proximal sensing line. An assisted breath is indicated by illumination of the assist/spontaneous LED.

The PLV-100 alarms in the event of low-pressure, high-pressure, apnea, inverse I:E ratio, low internal battery, low external battery, reverse battery connection, power failure, and ventilator malfunction. If the high-pressure setting is exceeded, the ventilator vents excess pressure. The PLV-100 can be powered from 12 volt or 110 household current and has an internal battery to power the unit in the event of power failure. An increased FIO_2 can be accomplished by adding oxygen to the inspiratory limb of the patient circuit.

The Lifecare PLV-102 (Figure 7.14) is an upgraded version of the PLV-100 with basically the same drive mechanism.

Sighs can be set to occur one out of every 100 volume limited breaths. During a sigh breath, the machine delivers 150% of the set tidal volume up to the maximum capabilities of the piston and cylinder (3,000 ml).

Oxygen is delivered by way of a proportioning valve dependent upon the tidal volume and oxygen percentage settings (Figure 7.15). The oxygen percentage in the inspiratory limb of the circuit is then monitored and corrected by the microprocessor if necessary to within 6%.[10] The effective oxygen percentage range that can be set is from 21–90%.[4]

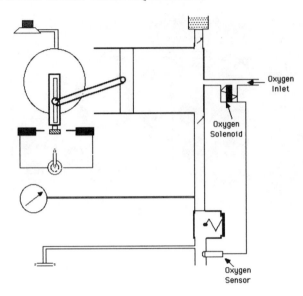

Oxygen
Inlet

Oxygen
Solenoid

Oxygen
Sensor

Figure 7.15 PLV-102 oxygen delivery system. Courtesy of Bear Medical Systems.

Indicators that have been added to the front panel include manual sigh, increased inspiratory flow rate, oxygen percentage, and alarm silence. The digital display that has been added is the alarm code which apears in the flowrate window.

The Puritan-Bennett Thompson M25A and M25B (Figures 7.16A & 7.16B) "Minilung" ventilators are piston driven and generate a sine wave flow pattern. Both units are capable of operation in the assist/control and control modes. The units can be modified to provide IMV with rates down to 4 breaths/minute with the addition of a bag type IMV system to the inspiratory leg of the patient circuit. The M25A was built into a Samsonite case and is no longer manufactured. The M25B, the current production model, is essentially the same ventilator, housed in an aluminum case. The motor and gear box move the piston in the cylinder in a rotary fashion. The rocker arm adjusts the piston stroke and therefore the volume delivered. The delivered volume is adjusted by shortening or lengthening the rocker arm. During the return stroke of the piston, gas is drawn into the cylinder through the inlet leaf valve. Once the piston returns to the end of the return stroke, an optical sensor is triggered, and current to the motor stops. The forward stroke begins either due to time (as determined by the rate control) in the case of a control breath, or by the patient triggering an assist breath. An assist breath is triggered by the patient's negative pressure drawing a diaphragm away from another optical sensor, which triggers current flow to the motor. During the forward stroke of the piston, gas exits the cylinder and flows past the pressure relief valve and onto through a one-way valve to the patient circuit. A smaller branch directs gas to the exhalation valve, occluding it during inspiration.

The tidal volume is adjustable from 300–2,500 ml and the rate is adjustable from 4–23 breaths/ minute. Inspiratory time is controlled by adjusting the current flow to the motor during inspiration and is adjustable from 1.3–5 seconds. The pressure-limit control adjusts the spring tension against the pop-off disc and can be adjusted from 10–70 cm H_2O pressure. The high pressure and low

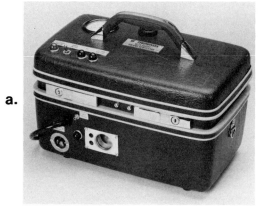

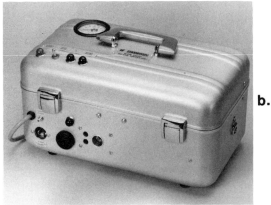

a.

b.

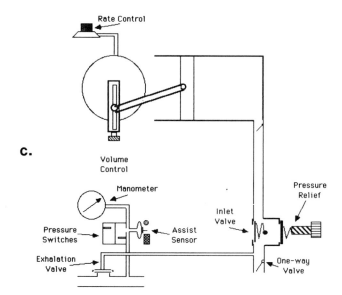

c.

Figure 7.16 **A** Puritan Bennett/Thompson M25A. Our grateful thanks to Puritan-Bennett's Portable Ventilator Division, Boulder, Colorado, for their assistance in helping us develop this material. **B** Puritan Bennett/Thompson M25B. Our grateful thanks to Puritan-Bennett's Portable Ventilator Division, Boulder, Colorado, for their assistance in helping us develop this material. **C** Bennett (Thompson) M25A & M25B schematic.

pressure alarms are factory pre-set at 65 and 12 cm H_2O pressure respectively. Adjustments to the pressure alarms can be made in the field, but should only be made by factory authorized service technicians.

The M25A has internal batteries capable of powering the ventilator for periods of 20–60 minutes in the event of a power failure. The M25B is capable of being powered by both 110 volt household current or a 12 volt car battery. Delivered oxygen percentages up to 50% can be obtained by the addition of an oxygen accumulator.

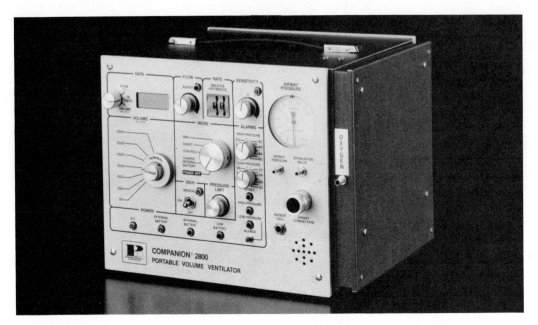

Figure 7.17 Puritan Bennett Companion 2800. Our grateful thanks to Puritan-Bennett's portable Ventilator Division, Boulder, Colorado, for their assistance in helping us develop this material.

In addition to the pressure alarms, the M25 has a low battery alarm. The exhalation valve has been criticized as having an allowable leak of up to 100 ml and for inadvertent improper assembly.[1]

The Puritan-Bennett Companion 2800 is a microprocessor controlled piston ventilator that produces a decelerating flow pattern (Figure 7.17). The Campanion 2800 can be operated in the control, assist/control, and SIMV modes. Manual and automatic sighs (three every 10 minutes) are available, with sigh volumes set on a separate sigh volume control. Tidal volumes are adjustable from 50–2,800 ml, and sigh volumes are adjustable from 125–2800 ml. The rate is adjustable from 1–69 breaths/minute and peak flows of 40–125 L/min are available.

The primary drive mechanism is similar to the drive mechanism for the M25, but functions in a different manner. A preset high pressure release is mounted directly on the piston itself, and fresh gas is drawn into the cylinder directly during the return stroke from an inlet in the head of the cylinder from a mixing chamber on the side of the unit (Figure 7.18). On the forward stroke of the piston, the current supplied to the motor is set by the flow control and determines the rate of piston travel and flow rate. The volume controls (normal and sigh) determine the distance that the piston travels during the forward stroke, in each mode of operation, and therefore sets the volume delivered. Gas exits the cylinder, past an adjustable peak pressure limit control and passes through the outlet one-way valve to the patient circuit. A smaller branch directs gas to the exhalation valve, inflating it during inspiration. Once the set distance has been traveled by the piston to deliver the set tidal volume, the polarity of the power to the motor is reversed, and the piston returns.

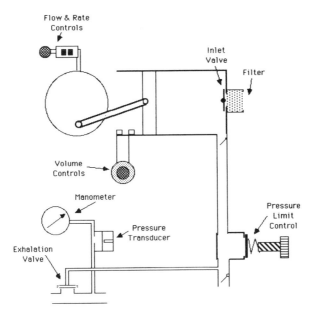

Figure 7.18 Bennett Companion 2800 schematic.

The sensitivity transducer senses patient effort through the proximal patient pressure line and is adjustable from -5 to $+15$ cm H_2O pressure. The pressure limit is adjustable from 10–70 cm H_2O pressure and the high pressure alarm range is 15–60 cm H_2O pressure. The low pressure alarm is adjustable from 2–32 cm H_2O pressure. A data display allows selection of digital display of peak flow, I:E, or volume. The alarm level is adjustable and a low pressure silence button silences the low pressure and apnea alarms for one minute.

Alarms on the 2800 include flow (inverse I:E of 1:0.8 or less), low pressure, high pressure, apnea (no patient effort for 15 seconds in SIMV), and low battery. If the patient fails to initiate a breath in SIMV for 45 seconds, the ventilator will switch to a back-up rate of 12 breaths/minute. A short audible alert occurs with a power change over and a malfunction of the ventilator causes a continous audible alarm. Remote alarm capabilities are available for the 2800 along with a patient activated call switch for the remote. Other indicators include power source, assisted breath, and sigh breaths.

The Bear 33 (Figure 7.19) volume ventilator is a microprocessor controlled, linear drive piston that is driven by a brushless motor and produces a sine wave flow pattern. Available modes include control, assist-control, SIMV, and sighs. The displacement and speed of the piston is controlled by the microprocessor to control delivered volume and flowrate. The available tidal volume range is 100–2,200 ml at a rates of 2–40 breaths/minute.[11] Inspiratory time can be varied from 0.25–5.0 seconds. The maximum peak pressure setting capability of the Bear 33 is 80 cm H_2O and a second internal safety over pressure release is set for 85 cm of H_2O. During SIMV, the patient draws the majority of gas from the gas accumulator directly through the cylinder by-pass valve (Figure 7.20). The accumulator is a maze of convolutions that act as a reservoir for oxygen accumulation. The delievered oxygen percentage can vary with changes in tidal volume and rate.

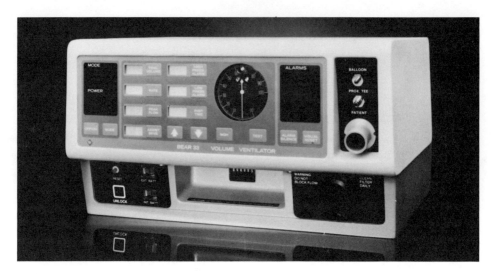

Figure 7.19 Bear 33 Ventilator. Courtesy of Bear Medical Systems, Riverside, CA.

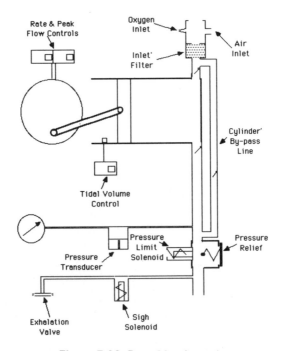

Figure 7.20 Bear 33 schematic.

Another source available to the patient is the cylinder itself, and room air can be drawn past the exhalation valve if a one-way valve is not placed on the valve outlet. Mandatory breath frequency is controlled by the rate control. When it is time for an assisted mandatory breath, the microprocessor opens an assist window that allows the patient to trigger a volume-limited, mandatory breath. In an effort to prevent stacking breaths, the assist window will not open for 750 milliseconds following a spontaneous or mandatory breath. A one-way valve on the exhalation valve outlet is recommended by the manufacturer to guarantee that leaks do not occur past the exhalation diaphragm during a patient assist effort. This could interfere with proper sensitivity of the assist sensor.

Sighs can be selected at a rate of 6/hour. When it is time for a sigh breath, the next assist effort or controlled rate breath on the part of the patient will trigger a sigh volume to be delivered. The Bear 33 will deliver 1.5 times the set tidal volume during a sigh breath with the capabilites of doing so up to a tidal volume set of 1,470 ml (a sigh volume of 2,190 ml) with one single stroke of the piston. With tidal volumes set higher than 1,470 ml, the sigh solenoid remains closed and the piston returns at maximum speed to deliver the remainder of the sigh breath with a second forward stroke (to a maximum sigh volume of 3,300 ml).

The Bear 33 is capable of selecting a power source in order of priority. The first priority is 110 volt household current, followed by an external 12 volt DC source. Finally, an internal battery can power the ventilator for up to one hour in the event of loss of the other external power sources. Both the internal and the external battery are charged when the ventilator is being powered by 110 volt AC current. Two selectable meters allow for checking the charge level of the internal and external batteries.

Audible and visual alarms on the Bear 33 include high-pressure, low-pressure, apnea, power source change, low internal battery and ventilator inoperative. There is also an audible complete power failure alarm. Digital diplays for tidal volume, rate, peak flow, assist sensitivity, high-pressure alarm, low-pressure alarm settings and for inspiratory time appear on the front panel of the Bear 33.

Bellows Ventilators

The Bennett MA-1 volume-limited ventilator (Figure 7.21) has been used in the home for many years. Originally designed for use in health care institutions, the MA-1 was selected for home care use because of its dependability, much as the Emerson Post-Op was choosen for this purpose.

Assist, assist-control, and IMV are possible with the MA-1. When inspiration is initiated, the main solenoid opens the flow of gas from the compressor to the jet of the venturi. The venturi entrains gas and the flow of air passes through a varible restrictor that adjusts the peak flow of gas from the venturi. The gas then flows to the bellows chamber, compressing the bellows upward, sending gas past the safety valve to the patient circuit. Another small line directs gas to the exhalation valve, inflating it during inspiration. When the bellows has reached a point determined by the tidal volume control, the main solenoid closes, stopping the flow of compressed air to the venturi. Flow from the venturi stops, and the bellows drops back to the bottom of the cylinder. As the bellows drops, gas is drawn in from the oxygen system. The oxygen system is essentially a

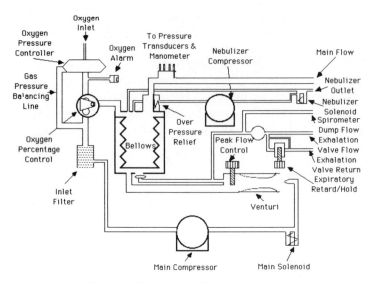

Figure 7.21 Bennett MA-1 schematic.

blender that operates at approximately atmospheric pressure. Oxygen supplied to the system is reduced to close to atmospheric pressure, and air pressure is balanced to the same pressure. Then the bellows draws a mixture of air and oxygen through a double, variable restrictor that determines the oxygen percentage delivered. As the oxygen percentage control is adjusted on the front panel, one orifice for air or oxygen is opened more while the other is closed more.

Tidal volumes can be set to 2,200 ml and the rate can be set from 6–60 breaths/minute. A modification for IMV allows the rate to be varied from less than 1 to as high as 60. The MA-1 delivers a tapering flow pattern.

During IMV, the patient draws gas from as optional demand valve or the standard H or bag IMV systems can be used. The rate control determines the delivery of the nonsynchronous volume delivered mandatory breaths.

One–three sighs are available at frequencies of 4, 6, 8, and 15 times per hour. The sigh volume is set on a separate sigh volume control and when it is time for a sigh breath to be delivered, the bellows rises to the level set by the sigh volume control. The cycle time for the ventilator is automatically doubled to allow longer exhalation time. A separate sigh pressure limit control allows the setting of a pressure limit different from that of the normal pressure limit. Both pressure limits have a range of up to 80 cm H_2O pressure.

Audiovisual alarms include high pressure, I:E ratio (less than 1:1, non-functional on assisted breaths), oxygen source loss alarm, and low tidal volume (with the optional monitoring spirometer). Visual indicators illuminate with assist effort and when a sigh breath(s) occur.

The MA-1 has the capabilities of adding varible expiratory resistance by partially occluding the flow of gas venting from the exhalation valve on expiration. The control is varible to the point of a short volume hold followed by maximum resistance to expiratory flow.

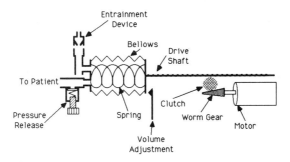

Figure 7.22 Pneumatic schematic for MVP 1500.

A nebulizer control provides a flow of gas on inspiration only, and draws its gas from the bellows so that neither oxygen percentage or delivered tidal volume is altered when a medication nebulizer isused.

A complete description of the MA-1 is found elsewhere.[3]

The Medimex MVP 1500 is a linear drive, bellows ventilator that produces a square wave flow pattern (Figure 7.22).

At the end of inspiration, a spring inside the bellows causes the bellows to inflate, drawing gas from the gas inlet (Figure 7.22). If oxygen concentrations higher that 21% are required, an entrainment device is attached to the gas inlet to supply the desired oxygen. Inspiration is initiated by the timing circuit of the rate control or by patient effort triggering the sensitivity transducer. The sensitivity is adjustable from −10 to 0 cm H_2O pressure, which functionally provides for assist, assist/control, and control and IMV modes. An electromagentic clutch engages and drives the bellows forward during inspiration, delivering gas to the patient and the exhalation valve. The tidal volume is set by adjusting the stopping point of the bellows during refill. Tidal volume is adjustable from 300–1,500 ml at rates of 4–18 breaths/minute. Once the bellows completes its forward travel, the electromagnetic clutch disengages, and the spring returns the bellows to the inflated position, refilling with gas from the entrainment device through the gas inlet. The rate of travel of the bellows is controlled by the inspiratory flow control. A screw type worm gear increases the speed of travel of the bellows with increases in inspiratory flow settings. Indicator lights display I:E ratios of 1:2 and whether the ratio is less than (shortage) or more than (extension) that value.

The high-pressure alarm can be adjusted to end inspiration between 20–70 cm H_2O pressure and the low-pressure alarm is adjustable from 5–50 cm H_2O pressure. An adjustable spring tension pressure release is mounted on the machine outlet.

The MVP 1500 is capable of being powered by household current, an external battery, or an internal battery that can power the ventilator for up to six hours for transport or in the event of power failure. Indicators on the front panel display the type of power source as well as an indication of charging of the battery. An internal battery check button allows checking the level of the internal battery.

Table 7.1   Specifications of Home Care Ventilators

	Modes	Tidal Volume Range	Rate Range	I:E	Pressure Limit/Cycle	Flow Pattern
Life Care PVV	Control	0–3,000	8–30	Fixed 1:1	100 Limit	Sine
Life Care PLV-100	C,A/C,SIMV	50–3,000	2–40	Variable	100 Cycle	Sine
Life Care PLV-102	C,A/C,SIMV	50–3,000	2–40	Variable	100 Cycle	Sine
Life Products LP-3	C,A/C	0–3,000	8–30	Fixed 1:1	100 Limit	Sine
Life Products LP-4	C/A/C,IMV	0–3,000	0.3–30	Fixed 1:1 Variable (A/C, 1MV)	100 Limit	Sine
Life Products LP-5	C,A/C,IMV	100–2,000	2–28	Variable	80 Cycle	Sine
Life Products LP-6	C,A/C,SIMV	100–2,000	1–38	Variable	100 Cycle	Decelerating
Bennett (Thompson) M25A&B	C,A/C	300–2,500	4–23	Variable	65 limit	Sine
Bennett Companion 2800	C,A/C,SIMV	50–2,800	1–69	Variable	70 Limit	Sine
Medimex MVP 1500	C,A/C, IMV	300–1,500		Variable		Square
Bear 33	C,A/C,SIMV	100–2,200	2–40	Variable	80 Cycle	Sine

References

1. Spearman C. B., Shelton R. L., Egan D. F. Egan's Fundamentals of respiratory therapy. 4th ed. St. Louis: The CV Mosby Co., 1982.
2. Burton G. G,, Hodgkin J. E., editors. Respiratory care: A guide to clinical practice. 2nd ed. Philadelphia: J.B. Lippincott Co., 1984.
3. McPherson S. P. Respiratory therapy equipment. 3rd ed. St. Louis: The C.V. Mosby Co., 1985.
4. Kacmarek R. M., Spearman C. B. Equipment used for ventilatory support in the home. Resp Care 1986; 31:1511.
5. Operational Manual, Model LP3 Volume Ventilator, LP3 OP. Boulder, CO: Life Products, Inc., 1984.

Oxygen Reservoir	Integral Oxygen Analyzer	Alarms									
		Pressure		Hc Limit	I:E	Flow	APNEA	Low Battery Power Loss	Alarm Silence	Remote Alarm	Patient Call
		Low	Hi								
No	No	Yes	Yes	No	No	No	No	Yes	No		
No	No	Yes	No	Yes	Yes	Yes	Yes	Yes	No		
Yes	Yes	Yes	No	Yes	Yes	Yes	Yes	Yes	Yes		
No	No	Yes	Yes	No	No	No	No	Yes	No		
No	No	Yes	Yes	No	No	No	Yes	Yes	No		
Yes	No	Yes	No	Yes	Yes	Yes	Yes	Yes	Yes		
Yes	No	Yes	No	Yes	Yes	No	Yes	Yes	Yes	Yes	
Yes	No	Yes	Yes	No	No	No	No	Yes	Yes		
Yes Added	No	Yes	Yes	No	Yes	Yes	Yes	Yes	No		Yes
Diluter	No	Yes	Yes	No	Yes	No		Yes	Yes		
Yes	No	Yes	No	Yes	Yes	Yes	Yes	Yes	Yes	Yes	

The above information was taken in part from, Kacmarek, R. M., and Spearman, C. B.: Equipment Used for Ventiliation Support in the Home, Respiratory Corp., April, 1986 3215.1. From manufacturer information on their products.

6. Operational Manual, Model LP4 Volume Ventilator, LP4 OP. Boulder, CO: Life Products, Inc., 1984.
7. Operational Manual, Model LP5 Volume Ventilator, LP5 OP. Boulder, CO: Life Products, Inc., 1984.
8. Users Guide and Instruction Manual, LP6 Compact Volume Ventilator, 70-65-001. Boulder, CO: Life Products, Inc., 1985.
9. Operating Manual, PLV-100, 35-500. Lafayette, CO: Lifecare, Inc., 1985.
10. Operating Manual, PLV-102, 37.500. Lafayette, CO: Lifecare, Inc., 1986.
11. Clinical Instruction Manual, Bear 33 Volume Ventilator, 50000-10133. Riverside, CA: Bear Medical Systems, Inc., 1984.

Appendix A

Company Directory

A

Abbey Medical/Abbey Rents, Inc.
3216 El Segundo Blvd.
Hawthorne, CA 90250
(213) 973–3493

Ackrad Laboratories, Inc.
70 Jackson Dr.
P.O. Box 1085
Cranford, NJ 07016
Bernard Ackerman
(201) 276–6390

Acucare Medical, Inc.
4155 E. Jewell Ave., Suite 602
Denver, CO 80222
Robert Thompson
(303) 759–8911

Advanced Instruments, Inc.
1000 Highland Ave.
Needham, MA 02194
R. V. Weston
(617) 449–3000

Aequitron Medical, Inc.
14130 23rd Avenue North
Minneapolis, MN 55441
Customer Service
(800) 824–7203
(612) 559–2012

Aeros Instruments, Inc.
3411 Commercial Ave.
Northbrook, IL 60062
Gordon D. Martin
(312) 272–8900

A & H Products, Inc.
P.O. Box 470854
Tulsa, OK 74147
Jerry Glenn
(918) 835–8081

Aimex Co., Inc.
114 State St.
Boston, MA 02109
Peter Thomson
(617) 227–7099

Airborne Life Support Systems
2409 N. Main
P.O. Box 77
Cleburne, TX 76031
John Segars
(817) 641–3385

Air Cleaning Specialists, Inc.
180 El Camino Real
Millbrae, CA 94030
J. C. Jordan
(415) 697–2761

Air-Shields/A Healthdyne Co.
330 Jackson Rd.
Hatboro, PA 19040
J. D. Miller
(800) 523–5756
In PA (800) 675–5200

Airlife/American Pharmaseal Company
27200 N. Tourney Rd.
Valencia, CA 91355–8900
Earl Roxran, Beth Elliott, Al Volk
(805) 253–1300

Air Products and Chemicals, Inc.
P.O. Box 538
Allentown, PA 18105
Paul A. Clydesdale
(215) 481–4911

Air Techniques, Inc.
1801 Whitehead Rd.
Baltimore, MD 21207
Sam Alima
(301) 944–6037

Alcide Corporation
One Willard Rd
Norwalk, CT 06851
(203) 847–2555

Alconox, Inc.
215 Park Ave. South
New York, NY 10003
W. Lebowitz
(212) 473–1300

ALKO Diagnostic Corp.
333 Fiske St., Alko Park
Holliston, MA 01746
(617) 429–4600

Allied Healthcare Products, Inc.
Chemetron Div.
1720 Sublette Ave.
St. Louis, MO 63110
John S. Martin
(314) 771–2400

Alpha Technologies, Inc.
3142-A Alcalde
Laguna Hills, CA 92653

Ambu Inc.
7 Old Sherman Tpk.
Danbury, CT 06810
Frank Homa
(800) AMBUINC
(203) 794–1221

Ambulatory Monitoring, Inc.
See Respitrace Corp.

Ambulatory Services of America
1800 Century Blvd., NE, Suite 780
Atlanta, GA 30345
Linda McCullough
(404) 321–4627

American Association for Respiratory Care (AARC)
1720 Regal Row, #112
Dallas, TX 75235
(214) 630–3540

Amerec Corp.
Health Care Products Div.
P.O. Box 3825
Bellevue, WA 98009
Lin Fassnacht
(800) 426–0858
(206) 643–1000

American Dade
Div. of American Hospital Supply Corp.
P.O. Box 520672
Miami, FL 33152
Robert W. Seitz
(305) 592–2311

American Edwards Labs
17221 Red Hill Ave.
Irvine, CA 92714
Allen Hill
(714) 250–2500

American Electromedics Corp.
13 Sagamore Park Rd.
Hudson, NH 03051
Sales/Marketing
(800) 343–0683
(603) 880–6300

American Health Products, Inc.
210 W. Main St., Suite 203
Tustin, CA 92680
(714) 669–9990
(800) 922–9990

American Hospital Supply Corp.
One American Plaza
Evanston, IL 60201
Vicki Bianchini
(312) 866–4000
(312) 473–0400

American Inhalation
P.O. Box 76128
Birmingham, AL 35223
Michael Gibran
(800) 633–3400

American Inhalation Representatives, Inc.
201 Beacon Pkwy. W.
Birmingham, AL 35209
Betsy Bass
(800) 633–3400

American Medical Alert Corp.
3265 Lawson Blvd.
Oceanside, NY 11572
(800) 645–3244
In NY (800) 632–6729

American Medical Development Corp.
251 University Dr.
Coral Gables, FL 33134
Alexander Tar
(305) 448–6821

American Optical Corp.
Eggert & Sugar Rds.
Buffalo, NY 14215
Andy Liberty
(716) 891–3000

American Pharmaseal Company
See Airlife/American Pharmaseal Co.

**American Scientific
    Products**
Div. of American Hospital
    Supply Corporation
General Offices
McGaw Park, IL 60085
(312) 689–8410

A–M Systems, Inc.
1220 75th St., SW
Everett, WA 98203
Ted McDonald
(800) 426–1306
(206) 353–1123

**Ametek/Thermox
    Instruments Division**
150 Freeport Rd.
Pittsburgh, PA 15238
Richard Wanek
(412) 828–9040

Analytical Products, Inc.
P.O. Box 845
Belmont, CA 94002
Ruth Holmes
(415) 592–1400

**HW Andersen Products,
    Inc.**
221 South St.
Oyster Bay, NY 11771
John Hamlin
(516) 922–5100

Anesthesia Associates, Inc.
460 Enterprise St.
San Marcos, CA 92069
George Jackson
(619) 744–6561

AO Scientific Instruments
P.O. Box 123
Buffalo, NY 14240
(716) 891–3000

Armac, Inc.
622 Route 10
Whippany, NJ 07981
James R. Bringard

**Armour Pharmaceutical
    Company**
303 South Broadway
Tarrytown, NY 10591
Steve Connelly
(914) 631–8888

Armstrong Industries, Inc.
3660 Commercial Ave.
P.O. Box 7
Northbrook, IL 60062
Warren G. Armstrong
(312) 272–5577
(800) 323–4220

Arvee, Inc.
730 E. Michigan Ave.
P.O. Box 460
Battle Creek, MI 49016
Duane M. Walters
(800) 537–9941
(616) 965–1423

ASF Co.
4570 S. Berkeley Lake Rd.
Norcross, GA 30071
Michael R. Meivers
(404) 441–3611

**Associated Distributors of
    Medical Devices, Inc.**
5373 NW 36 St., Suite 30
Miami, FL 33166
J. M. Alvarez
(305) 871–1940

**Astra Pharmaceutical
    Products, Inc.**
P.O. Box 1089
Framingham, MA 01701
Customer Service
(617) 620–0600

Audio-Digest Foundation
1577 E. Chevy Chase Dr.
Glendale, CA 91206
Kerry Herndon
(800) 423–2308

Avatron, Inc.
2970 Bay Vista Ct.
P.O. Box 429
Benecia, CA 94510
Rod Taylor
(707) 746–7800

Avery Laboratories, Inc.
145 Rome St.
Farmingdale, NY 11735
Abraham Chizik

AVL Scientific Corporation
33 Mansell Court
Roswell, GA 30077
Gerri Priest
(800) 526–2272
(404) 587–4040

Ayerst Laboratories
685 Third Ave.
New York, NY 10017
(212) 878–6043

B

B & F Medical Products, Inc.
P.O. Box 3656
1421 Expressway Dr. N.
Toledo, OH 43608
Jerry Knapp
(419) 729–0606

Baker's Medical
915 Divisadero St.
Fresno, CA 93721
Rick Krikorian
(209) 233–6063

Balston, Inc.
703 Massachusetts Ave.
P.O. Box C
Lexington, MA 02173
(800) 343–4048
(617) 861–7240

Bard-Parker
2 Bridgewater Lane
Lincoln Park, NJ 07035
Product Manager
(201) 628–9600
See ad on page 60

W.A. Baum Co., Inc.
620 Oak St.
Copiaque, NY 11726
James Baum
(516) 226–3940

Bay Corp.
867 Canterbury Rd.
Westlake, OH 44145
Sales Department
(216) 835–2212

Bear Medical Systems, Inc.
2085 Rustin Ave.
Riverside, CA 92507
(800) 331–2327
(714) 788–2460

Beckman Instruments, Inc.
See Sensormedics Corp.

Ben Venue Laboratories
Sterilant Division
270 Northfield Rd.
P.O. Box 46568
Bedford, OH 44146–0568
(800) 621–8848
(216) 232–3320

Benchmark Industries
1227 Colorado Ln.
Arlington, TX 76015
Don Humberd
(817) 460–1331

The Bendix Corp.
2734 Hickory Grove Rd.
P.O. Box 4508
Davenport, IA 52808
R. T. Lindsay
(319) 383–6000

Biochem International, Inc.
W238 N1650 Rockwood
Drive
Waukesha, WI 53188–1199
Alan H. Beder
(800) 558–2345
(414) 542–3100

Bio-Med Devices, Inc.
8 Bishop Lane
Madison, CT 96443
Dean Bennett
(203) 245–8765

BioMarine Industries, Inc.
45 Great Valley Center
Malvern, PA 19355
Billie Skolka
(215) 647–7200

**Bionaire Corporation/
BioMedisphere**
565A Commerce St.
Franklin Lakes, NU 07417
Anna Marie Licenziato
(201) 337–2110

Bio-Tek Instruments, Inc.
One Mill St.
Burlington, VT 05401
(800) 451–5172
In VT (800) 863–1880

Biotrine Corp.
52 Dragon St.
Woburn, MA 01801
(800) 245–8844
(617) 935–8844

Biox Technology, Inc.
See Ohmeda

Bird Products Corp.
3101 East Alejo Rd.
P.O. Box 2007
Palm Springs, CA 92263
Lisa Henke

Birtcher Corp.
Special Products Div.
4501 N. Arden Dr.
P.O. Box 4399
El Monte, CA 91734
Nancy Jensen
(213) 575–8144, ext. 242

Bivona Inc.
5700 West 23rd Ave.
Gary, IN 46406
Dolores Young
(219) 989–9150

**B–M Medical Products,
Inc.**
16318 W. Glendale Dr.
New Berlin, WI 53151
Mel Tates, Jr.
(414) 784–1511

**Boehringer Ingelheim
Pharmaceutical, Inc.**
90 East Ridge
Ridgefield, CT 06877

**Boehringer Laboratories,
Inc.**
P.O. Box 337
Wynnewood, PA 19096
(215) 642–4944

Robert J. Brady Co.
Routes 197 & 450
Bowie, MD 20715
Edie Plunkett
(301) 262–6300

Brentwood Instruments
3425 Lomita Blvd.
Torrance, CA 90505
Richard Rosenthal
(800) 624–8950

Briox Technologies, Inc.
93 Grand St.
Worchester, MA 01610
Customer Service Dept.
(800) 225–7496

Howard Bruce Co.
17330 Burbank Blvd.,
No. 9
Encino, CA 91316
Howard Bruce
(213) 986–8273

BSL Technology
5060 W. Amelia Earhart
Dr.
Salt Lake City, UT 84116
(801) 355–7100

**Buffalo Medical Specialties
Mfg. Inc. (BMS)**
14205 Myerlake Circle
Clearwater, FL 33520
John Garrett
(800) 237–8937

The John Bunn Co.
290 Creekside Dr.
Tonawanda, NY 14150
Joe Marciano
(800) 828–7331

Burnishine Products
8140 Ridgeway Ave.
Skokie, IL 60076
(312) 583–1810

C

**California College for
Health Sciences**
1810 State St.
San Diego, CA 92101
Edward C. Moser
(619) 232–3488

CalTech Industries, Inc.
217 E. Main St.
P.O. Box 1139
Midland , MI 48640
C. N. Goeders
(517) 636–7700

Cardionics, Inc.
15502 Old Galveston Rd.
Suite 220
Webster, TX 77598
Keith Johnson
(713) 488–5901

Cardionostics, Inc.
1562 Parkway Loop
Tustin, CA 92680
Mike Halverson
(714) 259–1582

Catalyst Research
3706 Crondall Ln.
Owings Mill, MD 21117
Bob Kalish
(800) 851–4500

Cavitron Cardiopulmonary
270 E. Palais Rd.
Anaheim, CA 92805
Gary Prickett
(800) 854–3894
(714) 776–1811

CDX Corp.
10691 E. Bethany Dr., #900
Aurora, CO 80014
Sales Mgr.
(800) 525–3515
(303) 695–8751

Centronic
King Henry's Dr.
New Addington
Croydon CR9 OBG
U.K.

Chad Therapeutics, Inc.
9749 Independent Ave.
Chatsworth, CA 91311
Frank R. Fleming
(800) 423–8870
(818) 882–0883

Charter Laboratories
P.O. Box 1774
Toms River, NJ 08753
Ray Bonthron
(201) 367–2300

Chemetron
See Allied Healthcare
    Products

Chesebrough-Pond's, Inc.
33 Benedict Place—
    Glenville
Greenwich, CT 06830
J. Biondo
(203) 625–2210

Chestech Corp.
See SensorMedics Corp.

**Ciba Corning Diagnostics
    Corp.**
63 North St.
Medfield, MA 02052
(800) 255–8769

**Ciba Medical Education
    Div.**
556 Morris Ave.
Summit, NJ 07901
Ward Newschwander
(201) 277–5058

**Clean Air Work Stations,
    Inc.**
P.O. Box 50
Commack, NY 11725
(516) 543–0327

**Clinical Data Instruments,
    Inc.**
P.O. Box 430
Brookline, MA 02146
Phil Lang
(617) 734–3700

Cloud 9
Div. of Mason Engineering
    Corp.
242 West Devon Ave.
Bensenville, IL 60106
Jon E. Spranger
(312) 595–5700

Colgate Palmolive Co.
300 Park Ave.
New York, NY 10022
Frank P. Corso
(212) 751–1200, ext. 342

Warren E. Collins, Inc.
220 Wood Rd.
Braintree, MA 02184
Sales Dept.
(617) 843–0610

**Computer Instruments
    Corp.**
100 Madison Ave.
Hempstead, NY 11550
Burton H. Birnbaum
(800) 227–1314
(516) 483–8200

Concord Labs
Kit St.
Keene, NH 03431
R. Michael Weldon

Corning Medical
See Ciba Corning
    Diagnostics Corp.

**Corometrics Medical
    Systems, Inc.**
61 Barnes Park Rd. North
Wallingford, CT 06492
Mike Tuccio
(800) 243–3952
(203) 265–5631

**Corpak Respiratory
    Therapy**
140 W. Hintz Rd.
Wheeling, IL 60090
(800) 323–6305
(312) 537–4601

Corpul Metrix, Inc.
6415 SW Canyon Ct., Suite
    50
Portland, OR 97221
Toni Schubert
(503) 297–3383

Crest Ultrasonics Corp.
Scotch Rd.
Trenton, NJ 08628
Marvin S. Detwiler
(800) 441–9675
(609) 883–4000

Critikon, Inc.
P.O. Box 22800
Tampa, FL 33630
Customer Service
(800) 237–7541
In FL (800) 282–9151

Cryogenic Associates
6565 Coffman Rd.
P.O. Box 687710
Indianapolis, IN 46268
Sales Department
(317) 298–7333

Cryomed Corp.
P.O. Box 2078
Ft. Pierce, FL 33454
Doug Hatton
(800) 327–0313
(305) 465–6660

Cryo₂ Corp.
P.O. Box 2078
4106 Ave. D
Ft. Pierce, FL 33454
Robert W. McCoy
(800) 327–0313
(305) 465–6660

Cura Care
550A Western Dr.
Mobile, AL 36609
Bill Jackson
(205) 476–7950

**Current Reviews in
Respiratory Therapy, Inc.**
1200 NW Tenth Ave.
Miami, FL 33136

Current Technologies, Inc.
P.O. Box 21
Crawfordsville, IN 47933
Tom Goch
(317) 364–0490

**Curtin Matheson Scientific,
Inc.**
P.O. Box 1546
Houston, TX 77251
Cecil Kost
(713) 820–1661

Cutter Resiflex
1630 Industrial Park St..
Covina, CA 91722
Doug Keasling
(213) 339–7388

D

Dale Medical Products, Inc.
7 Cross St.
P.O. Box 1556
Plainville, MA 02762
Daniel W. McElaney
(800) 343–3980
(617) 695–9316

Dart Respiratory
See Seamless Hospital
Products, Inc.

Datamatic Services
200 Windsor Dr.
Oak Brook, IL 60521
Donna Stuben
(312) 654–1810

Datascope Corporation
580 Winters Ave.
P.O. Box 5
Paramus, NJ 07653–0005
O. Arnay
(201) 265–8800

Datamed Corporation
4029 Knight Arnold Rd.
Memphis, TN 38118
Adele P. Kissinger
(901) 363–3688

**Davco Chemicals and
Plastics, Inc.**
See Medical Molding Corp.
of America

**F. A. Davis Company,
Publishers**
1915 Arch St.
Philadelphia, PA 19103–
1493
James C. Mills
(215) 568–2270

Deltech Engineering, Inc.
Century Park, P.O. Box 667
New Castle, DE 19720
Russ Goldsmith
(302) 328–1345

The Deseret Co.
9450 S. State St.
Sandy, UT 84070
Clem Fullmor
(801) 255–6851

**DeVilbiss Health Care
Worldwide**
P.O. Box 635
Somerset, PA 15501–0635
(800) 433–1331
(814) 443–4881

Dey Laboratories, Inc.
10246 Miller Rd.
Dallas, TX 75238
Duane L. Young
(800) 527–4278
(214) 349–7275

DHD Medical Products,
Division of Diemolding
Corp.
125 Rasbach St.
Canastota, NY 13032
Ron McHenry
(800) 847–8000
(315) 697–2221

Diatek, Inc.
3910 Sorrento Valley Blvd.
San Diego, CA 92121
Customer Service
(800) 854–2904

**Diverse Respiratory
Air Products**
570 W. Terrace Way
San Dimas, CA 91773
Dave Richard
(714) 599–0975

Dixie USA, Inc.
P.O. Box 13060
Houston, TX 77219
(800) 231–6230
In TX (800) 392–4335

DNA Medical, Inc.
3385 West 1820 South
Salt Lake City, UT 84104
Gregory A. Miller, Jr.
(801) 973–4600

**Dow Infection
Control Products**
P.O. Box 11339
Midland, Ml 48640
(517) 636–1000

Dryden Corp.
P.O. Box 36038
10640 E. 59th St.
Indianapolis, IN 46236
Customer Service
(800) 428–5321
(317) 823–6866

Duralast Products Corp.
100 Napoleon Ave.
New Orleans, LA 70130
Jack Rich, Jr.
(504) 895–2068

Dwyer Precision Inc.
266 North 20th St.
P.O. Box 51182
Jacksonville Beach, FL
32250
P. W. Dwyer
(904) 249–3545

E

Eastern Anesthesia, Inc.
1448 Ford Rd.
Bensalem, PA 19020
James A. Gunnerson
(215) 639–7880

Eastern Rail Systems Inc.
15 Friends Lane
Newtown, PA 18940
James A. Gunnerson
(215) 639–7880

**Eastern Respiratory
Services, Inc.**
35-35 E. Fifth St.
Mt. Carmel, PA 17851
David Horsfield
(717) 339–4000

Ecology Tech
P.O. Box 1598
Jonesboro, AR 72401
Bill Bobbitt
(501) 932–6262

EDL Corp.
417 Wakara Way
Salt Lake City, UT 84108
Robert L. Springmeyer Jr.
(801) 582–0515

**Education Resource
Consortium, Inc.**
190 E. Sweetbriar Dr.
Claremont, CA 91711
(714) 621–6261

Elder Oxygen Co., Inc.
4848 Ronson Ct., Suite G
San Diego, CA 92111
(714) 560–1991

**ElectroCardioGram
Systems**
(ECG Systems)
550A Western Dr.
Mobile, AL 36607
Bill Jackson
(205) 476–7950

Electronic Monitors, Inc.
P.O. Box 1087
Euless, TX 76039
Roger Siverson
(817) 283–0859

Eltron Corp., Airomax Div.
1941 Old Cuthbert Rd.
Cherry Hill, NJ 08034
Joseph Mogur
(609) 428–3311

J. H. Emerson Co.
22 Cottage Park Ave.
Cambridge, MA 02140
(800) 252–1414
(617) 864–1414

Empire Medical Products
6588 Daveson Blvd.
Norcross, GA 30093
Steve Walker
(404) 488–1113

**Encyclopaedia Britannica
Educational Corp.**
425 North Michigan Ave.
Chicago, IL 60611
Customer Relations
(800) 345–1136
In PA call collect
(214) 687–5544

Energen Products Co.
P.O. Box 45222
Dallas, TX 75245
Gary Nelson
(214) 241–8252

Equilibrated Bio Systems, Inc.
900 Watt Whitman Rd.
Melville, NY 11747
Alex Stenzler
(516) 673–6660

Equimed Equipment, Inc.
700 Waverly Ave., P.O. Box 362
Mamaroneck, NY 10543
Alan J. Landauer
(914) 698–6500

Erie Medical
4000 South 13th St.
Milwaukee, WI 53221
Robert Rakers
(414) 747–7022

Erie Medical (Canada) LTD.
P.O. Box 880
Stouffville, Ontario L0H 1L0
(416) 640–2363

Essex Industries, Inc.
7700 Gravois Ave.
St. Louis, MO 63123
(314) 832–4500
Telex 44–2310

Esterline Angus Instrument Corp.
P.O. Box 24000
Indianapolis, IN 46224
(317) 244–7611

Everest & Jennings, Inc.
3233 E. Mission Oaks Blvd.
Camarill, CA 93010
Dou Donnalley
(805) 987–6911

ExperCorp. Inc.
4065 West Charleston Blvd.,
Suite 200
Las Vegas, NV 89102
William T. McGee
(702) 877–1733

Exidyne Bio-Medical Technologies, Inc.
1229 Lake Plaza Dr.
Colorado Springs, CO 80906
(303) 576–3700

Extracorporeal Medical Specialties
See Critikon, Inc.

F

Fairfield Medical Products
845 East Main St.
Stamford, CT 06902
Ruth P. Newell
(203) 357–1855

W. T. Farley, Inc.
4450 Shopping Lane
Simi Valley, CA 93063
Rose D. Sigman
(800) FARLEYS
(805) 526–4991
(818) 999–4244

Ferraris Medical, Inc.
9681 Wagner Rd.
Holland, NY 14080
Dave Malys
(716) 537–2391

Fisher Scientific Co.
711 Forbes Ave.
Pittsburgh, PA 15219
(412) 562–8339

Fisher & Paykel Medical, Inc.
Northway Plaza
Upper Glen St.
Glens Falls, NY 12801
(518) 793–2155

International Office
Auckland, New Zealand
Telex 791–2985Z

Fiske Med-Science
See Med-Science

Fisons Corp.
2 Preston Ct.
Bedford, Ct.
Bedford, MA 01730
(617) 275–1000, ext 254

Flintrol, Inc
3521 Airport Rd.
P.O. Box 1598
Jonesboro, AR 72401
E. C. Nicholson
(800) 643–0000
(501) 932–6262

Fogg System Company, Inc.
15592 E. Batavia Dr.
Aurora, CO 80011
(800) 525–0292
(303) 344–1883

The Foredom Electric Co.
Route 6
Bethel, CT 06801
Kent Kristensen
(203) 792–8622

Foregger Medical
Div. of Puritan-Bennett
   Corp.
835 Wheeler Way
P.O. Box 550
Langhome, PA 19047
Michael L. Murphy
(215) 752-9405

Fraser Harlake Inc.
145 Mid County Dr.
Orchard Park, NY 14127
Regional Customer Service
   Reps.
(716) 662-6650

FutureMed
Division of Future Impex
   Corp.
2076 Deer Park Ave.
Deer Park, NY 11729
Morad Davoudzadeh
(516) 242-1616

G

Gambro, Inc.
Engstrom Division
600 Knights Bridge Pkwy.
Lincolnshire, IL 60069
Customer Service
(312) 634-6411

Gast Manufacturing Corp.
P.O. Box 97
Benton Harbor, MI 49022
(616) 926-6171

Gaymar Industries, Inc.
10 Centre Dr.
Orchard Park, NY 14127
L. L. Wolgemuth
(800) 828-7341
(716) 662-2551

**General Biomedical Service,
   Inc.**
7060 Read Lane, Suite 103
New Orleans, LA 70127
William Dwyer
(504) 241-1841

General Diagnostics
Div. of Warner-Lambert
201 Tabor Rd.
Morris Plains, NJ 07950
(800) 631-8060

General Physiotherapy, Inc.
1520 Washington Ave.
St. Louis, MO 63103
Timothy Chance
(314) 231-9643

Giaxco, Inc.
1900 W. Commercial Blvd.
Ft. Lauderdale, FL 33309
David Wright

Gomco Division
See Allied Healthcare
   Products, Inc.

Gould, Inc.
Cardiopulmonary Products
   Div.
805 Liberty Lane
Dayton, OH 45449
Ovid L. Bailey
(800) 543-9438
(513) 859-9000
Telex 205-444

Greene & Kellogg
290 Creekside Dr.
Tonawanda, NY 14150
(716) 691-7474

**Grundy Environmental
   Systems, Inc.**
3939 Raffin Rd.
San Diego, CA 92123
(619) 278-6500

**Gulf States Computer
   Services, Inc.**
10039 Bissonnet, Suite 130
Houston, TX 77036
George R. Foster
(713) 270-9003

H

Hamilton Medical, Inc.
4980 Energy Way
P.O. Box 30008
Reno, NV 89520
G. Eric Gjerde
(702) 786-7599

Hankscraft by Gerber
728 Rooster Blvd.
P.O. Box 120
Reedsburg, WI 53959
(608) 524-4341

Harris Calorific
Div. of Emerson Electric
   Co.
400 Clark St.
Elyria, OH 44036
Phil Preuninger
(216) 961-5700

Haskel, Inc.
Engineered Products Div.
100-76 E. Graham Pl.
Burbank, CA 91502
Victor Aello
(213) 843-4000

H.B. Laboratories, Inc.
16 Yankee Peddler Path
Madison, CT 96443
Dean J. Bennett
(203) 245–4972

**Health Technology
  Laboratories, Inc.**
Wissahickon Ave. at
  Dickerson Rd.
P.O. Box 1097
North Wales, PA 19454
(800) 345–4081
(215) 699–8787

Healthdyne, Inc.
2253 Northwest Parkway
Marietta, GA 30067
Customer Service
(404) 955–9555

Healthmark Industries Co.
22522 E. Nine Mile Rd.
St. Clair Shores, MI 48080
Ralph A. Basile
(800) 521–6224
(313) 774–7760

HealthScan Products, Inc.
908 Pompton Ave.
Cedar Grove, NJ 07009
Purchasing Department
(800) 962–1266
(201) 239–3139

Herco Products Inc.
P.O. Box 2903
Toledo, OH 43606
W. Walters
(419) 535–7490

Hewlett-Packard
100 Fifth Avenue
Waltham, MA 02254
Contact local sales office

**High Stoy Technological
  Corp.**
160 Wilbur Pl.
Bohemia, NY 11716
Lee Hadin
(516) 589–8900

Honeywell, Inc.
Biomedical Equipment
  Service
4800 E. Dry Creek Rd.
Denver, CO 80217
(303) 771–4700
Service Only

Honeywell, Inc.
TID Instrumentation
  Services
P.O. Box 5227
Denver, CO 80217
Richard Janes
(303) 771–4700

Hospal Medical Corp.
4100 E. Dry Creek Rd.
Littleton, CO 80122
Jeff Butler
(303 770–2700

Hospitak, Inc.
1144 Rte. 109
Lindenhurst, NY 11757
(800) 634–6003
Customer Service

**Hospital Pulmonary
  Services**
P.O. Box 92
Modesto, CA 95353
(209) 521–2330

HR Inc.
P.O. Box 1744
Bellevue, WA 98009
(800) 426–1042
(206) 881–7761

Hudson Oxygen
27711 Diaz Street
P.O. Box 66
Temecula, CA 92390–0066
Thomas C. Loescher
(800) 521–0748
In CA (800) 221–0338

Orange Park, FL
56 Industrial Loop
P.O. Box 555
32073–0555
(800) 362–6783
In FL (800) 342–0183
Wadsworth, OH
2106 Seville Rd.
P.O. Box 1000, 44281–0901
(800) 392–7252
In OH (800) 367–8783

Humetrics Corp.
353 N. Oak St.
Inglewood, CA 90302
(213) 673–3002

**Huntington Laboratories,
  Inc.**
970 E. Tipton St.
Huntington, IN 46750
Manager, Customer Service
(219) 356–8100

Hyrex Pharmaceuticals
P.O. Box 18385
3494 Democrat Rd.
Memphis, TN 38118
Jones or Baker
(901) 794–9050

I

IADEC
1A Lincoln Ave.
Albany, NY 12205
Harold Tomlinson
(518) 869–3240

IBM Corp.
P.O. Box 10
Princeton, NJ 08540
Irene Joyce

Ideal Medical
Div. of Puritan-Bennett
  Corp.
5805 Millett Hwy.
Lansing, MI 48917
(517) 322–9500

ILC Dover
P.O. Box 266
Frederica, DE 19946
Rhonda Ksionek
(302) 335–3911

Impact Medical Corp.
Leonia Ave.
P.O. Box 412
Bogota, NJ 07603
Michael Peluso
(201) 343–3004

InfaWatch
4000 MacArthur Blvd.
Suite 3000
Newport Beach, CA 92660
(714) 666–0395

Infomed Corporation
13 Inverness Way South
Englewood, CO 80112
Paul W. Shatusky
(303) 790–1311

Infrasonics, Inc.
9944 Barnes Canyon Rd.
San Diego, CA 92121
Guy Gansel
(619) 450–9898

Inhalation Plastics Inc.
7790 N. Merrimac
Niles, IL 60648
Robert A. Faber
(312) 763–3600

Inhalation Therapy Service
4 Militia Dr.
Lexington, MA 02173
Jeff Byer
(617) 861–8950

Inspiron Corporation
A Subsidiary of Omnicare,
  Inc.
8600 Archibald Avenue
Rancho Cucamonga, CA
  91730
Cheryl Vasquez
(714) 980–0088

**Instasan Pharmaceuticals,
  Inc.**
12850 Lyndon Ave.
Detroit, MI 48227
Dean Tabin
(800) 521–8100
(313) 935–3300

**Instrumentation Industries,
  Inc.**
2990 Industrial Blvd.
Bethel Park, PA 15102
Edward C. Horey, Jr.
(412) 854–1133

**Instrumentation Laboratory,
  Inc.**
113 Hartwell Ave.
Lexington, MA 02173
(800) 225–4040

Intec Medical, Inc.
22200 East 40 Hwy.
Blue Springs, MO 64015
Joe Brown
(800) 821–8598

Intercoastal Leasing Group
1299 Fourth St.
San Rafael, CA 94901
Art Wald

InterMetro Industries Corp.
North Washington St.
Wilkes-Barre, PA 18705
John G. Nackley
(717) 825–2741

**International Biomedical,
  Inc.**
2409 N. Main
P.O. Box 77
Cleburne, TX 76031
(817) 641–3385

**International Concordium,
  Inc.**
5171 Douglas Fir Rd.
Calabasas, CA 91302
Dennis Schwesinger
(213) 702–0502

Invacare Corp.
899 Cleveland St.
P.O. Box 4028
Elyria, OH 44036–2125
(800) 362–5715
In OH (800) 362–7415

Isothermal/American Pharmaseal Company
333 Durahart St.
Riverside, CA 92507
Al Volk, Joyce Roeder
(714) 686–8900

IT & E Inc.
10723 White Oak Ave.
Granada Hills, CA 91343
(213) 894–4116

J

Erich Jaeger, Inc.
5251 Zenith Pkwy.
Rockford, IL 61111–2728
Ron Evenson
(800) THE-LUNG
(815) 633–6400

Johnson & Johnson
501 George St. #J306
New Brunswick, NJ 08903
Frederick Gammon

Jones Medical Instrument Co.
200 Windsor Dr.
Oak Brook, IL 60521
Donna Stuben
(312) 654–1810

K

K & G Health Care Industries, Inc.
5373 N.W. 36th St. Suite 4
Miami Springs, FL 33166
Erik E. Berg
(305) 871–3632

Kay Laboratories, Inc.
P.O. Box 81471
San Diego, CA 92001
Customer Service
(714) 297–5470

Kaz Inc.
10 Columbus Circle
New York, NY 10019
(212) 586–1630

Key Pharmaceuticals, Inc.
P.O. Box 693670
18425 N.W. Second Ave.
Miami, FL 33269
(305) 652–2276

Kinetic Concepts
3417 Steen Dr.
San Antonio, TX 78219
James E. Toombs
(512) 225–4092

Kinetics Measurement Co.
118 Rt. 17 N. Marron Park
Upper Saddle River, NJ 07458
Dick Toomey

King Systems Corporation
15015 Herriman Blvd.
Noblesville, IN 46060
Kevin Burrow

Kontron Instruments
9 Plymouth St.
Everett, MA 02149
Alison Pena
(617) 389–6400

L

Laerdal Medical Corp.
1 Labriola Court
Armonk, NY 10504
John W. Reilly
(800) 431–1055

Laminar Flow, Inc.
102 Richard Rd.
Ivyland, PA 18974
Sales Dept.
(215) 672–0232

Larson Laboratories, Inc.
1320 Irwin Dr.
Erie, PA 16505
(814) 452–6815

Lea & Febiger
600 South Washington Sq.
Philadelphia, PA 19106–4198
Customer Service
(800) 433–3850
(215) 922–1330

LeMans Industries Corp.
225 Grand St.
Brooklyn, NY 11211
Harry Mandler
(516) 997–9071

Lexington Instrument Corp.
221 Crescent St.
Waltham, MA 02154
Ken Grooper
(617) 899–0410

Lifecare
5505 Central Ave.
Boulder, CO 80301
Janice K. Campbell
(303) 443–9234

Lifeguard Medical Products
6212 S. Fairfield Road
Indianapolis, IN 46241
Jay Hayes
(317) 248–8068

**Lifemark Ancillary
  Services, Inc.**
P.O. Box 3448
Houston, TX 77001
Sales
(713) 621–8131

LifeMed Technologies, Inc.
8630 Westpark Dr.
Houston, TX 77063
(800) LIFEMED
(713) 952–0500

Life Products, Inc.
2545 Central Ave.
Boulder, CO 80301
Bob Mallory
(303) 444–7606

Lif-O-Gen
Div. of U.S. Diver Co.
P.O. Box 149
Woods Rd.
Cambridge, MD 21613
Frank Pytryga or
Warren Newcomb
(800) 638–1197
(301) 228–6400

Life Support Products, Inc.
P.O. Box 19569
Irving, CA 92713
Kim Golemb
(714) 859–0777

Lippincott/Harper
E. Washington St.
Philadelphia, PA 19105
John Ranonis

Liquid Air Corp.
P.O. Box 149, Woods Rd.
Cambridge, MD 21613
Richard F. O'Brien
(800) 638–1197

Liquid Carbonic Corp.
135 South LaSalle St.
Chicago, IL 60603
R. K. Panaras
(312) 855–2500

Little, Brown and Co.
Medical Div.
34 Beacon St.
Boston, MA 02106
Customer Service
(617) 227–0730

Litton Datamedix
Route One
Sharon, MA 02067
(800) 225–0455
In MA (800) 532–9683

Litton Medical Electronics
See Litton Datamedix

Lorenz Instruments
638 29th Ave.
San Francisco, CA 94121
Henry R. Lorenz
(415) 386–7544

LSE Corp.
Div. of Puritan-Bennett
  Corp.
6 Gill St.
Woburn, MA 01801
Charles W. Frederico
(617) 935–4954

Lung Care, Inc.
P.O. Box 545
Cudahy, WI 53110
(414) 681–0111

Luxfer USA, LTD
P.O. Box 56100
Riverside, CA 92517
J. R. Ament
(714) 684–5110

M

**Mada Medical Products,
  Inc.**
60 Commerce Rd.
Carlstadt, NJ 07072
Dr. Ralph A. Adam
(210) 460–0454

Mallinckrodt Critical Care
Div. Mallinckrodt, Inc.
73 Quaker Rd.
Glens Falls, NY 12801
Sandy McIntosh
(800) 833–8842
In NY (800) 342–4010
(518) 793–6671

**Marathon Medical
  Equipment Corp.**
6703 A East 47th Ave. Dr.
Denver, CO 80216
John R. Porter
(800) 525–0654

Marion Laboratories
10236 Bunker Ridge Rd.
Kansas City, MO 64137
(800) 821–7313

**Marquest Medical
    Products, Inc.**
11039 Lansing Circle
Englewood, CO 80112
Thomas H. Miller
(303) 790–4835

Marquette Electronics, Inc.
8200 West Tower Avenue
Milwaukee, WI 53223
Monitoring: Tom Divers
Diagnostics, ECG, and
    Stress: John Lovett
(414) 355–5000

Marshall Electronics, Inc.
5425 W. Fargo Ave.
Skokie, IL 60077
(312) 674–6100

Martech, Inc.
Airport Office Center, 2B
Latrobe, PA 15650
Gary J. Turnbull
(412) 539–3130

Martell Medical
7555 Jurupa Ave., Suite E
Riverside, CA 92504
Michael D. Martell
(800) 624–9400
(714) 359–7780
(714) 359–7783

Marx Medical, Inc.
5660 LaJolla Blvd.
La Jolla, CA 92037
(714) 453–0351

Masterseal Medical Corp.
1621 Collingwood Dr.
San Diego, CA 92109
Wallace Hall

McGinnis Enterprises
1370 Brea Blvd., Suite 230
Fullerton, CA 92635
(714) 870–1760

MD Software, Inc.
1675 North D St.
San Bernardino, CA 92405
(714) 883–3019

Mead Johnson
Pharmaceutical Div.
2404 W. Pennsylvania St.
Evansville, IN 47721

Medcom, Inc.
P.O. Box 116
Garden Grove, CA 92641
(800) 854–2485
In CA (800) 472–2479

**Medical Engineering
    Corporation**
3037 Mt. Pleasant St.
Racine, WI 53404
David Monnot
(800) 558–9494

**Medical Equipment
    Designs, Inc.**
23521 Ridge Route Dr.,
    Suite A
Laguna Hill, CA 92653
(800) 323–1674
(714) 859–7779

Medical Graphics Corp.
350 Oak Grove Pkwy.
St. Paul, MN 55126
Kye A. Anderson
(612) 484–4874
(800) 328–4138

**Medical Instrumentation
    Brokers, Inc.**
3750 NW 28th St. #309
Miami, FL 33142
Elias K. Artze
(800) 327–4477

Medical IntelCom Inc.
2810 W. Charleston,
Suite H-82
Las Vegas, NV 89102
(702) 877–1733

**Medical Molding
    Corporation of America**
240 Briggs Ave.
Costa Mesa, CA 92626
Terry Bagwell
(714) 546–4161

**Medical Plastics
    Laboratory, Inc.**
P.O. Box 38
Gatesville, TX 76528
H. T. Jenkins
(800) 433–5539

Medical Specifics, Inc.
4418 Sunbolt Dr.
Dallas, TX 75248
Judy Chilton
(800) 437–PUMP
(214) 931–7569

Medical Systems
2580 Arizona Ave., #8
Santa Monica, CA 90404

Medicon, Inc.
See Aequitron Medical,
    Inc.

Medicor, Inc.
1559 E. Stratford Ave.
Salt Lake City, UT 84119
(801) 486–0121

**Mediq/PRN Life Support
Services, Inc.**
One Mediq Plaza
Pennsauken, NJ 08110
Lee F. Weiler, Jr.
(800) 257–7477
In NJ (800) 232–6960
(609) 665–8890

Medimex, Inc
300 Hempstead Tpke.
West Hempstead, NY
  11552
(516) 292–3375
Telex 645–225 Medimex
  Hemp

Medix Limited
Medix House
Main St.
Catthorpe, Lutterworth,
Leicestershire, LE17 6DB
England
Philip G. Stimpson
Telex 342254 Tango G.

Med-Science
1455 Page Industrial Blvd.
St. Louis, MO 63132
Dorothy Jovaag
(800) 325–4830
(314) 427–1000

MEM Medical, Inc.
271 Cleveland Ave.
Highland Park, NJ 08904
Customer Service
(201) 249–2880

Mercury Enterprises, Inc.
P.O. Box 20000
St. Petersburg, FL 33742
Garry P. Blount
(813) 576–4985

MES Inc.
3041 N. California St.
Burbank, CA 91504
Customer Service
(800) 423–2215
(818) 846–4343

Metrex Research Corp.
P.O. Box 965
11270 S. Dransfeldt Rd.
Parker, CO 80134
(303) 841–5842

**Metropolitan Wire
Corporation**
See InterMetro Industries
  Corporation

**Michigan Lake Medical
Products**
718 Simpson St.
Kalamazoo, MI 49007
Hawley Forde
(616) 345–4824

Micro Analytic Co.
P.O. Box 21
Crawfordsville, IN 47933
Tom Goch
(317) 364–0490

**Mill-Rose Laboratories,
Inc.**
8141 Tyler Blvd.
Mentor, OH 44060
Mark Kozak, Bev Gordon
(800) 321–1380
(216) 255–7995

**Mistogen Equipment
Company**
See The Timeter Group

MKS Instruments, Inc.
34 Third Ave.
Burlington, MA 01803
Grant Armstrong
(617) 272–9255

**Modern Engineering Co.
Inc.**
P.O. Box 14858
St. Louis, MO 63178
James F. Fausek
(800) 325–8178

Monaghan Medical Corp.
Route 9 N., Franklyn Bldg.
Plattsburgh, NY 12901
Michael T. Amato
(518) 561–7330

**P. K. Morgan Instruments,
Inc.**
Two Dundee Park, Level 1
Andover, MA 01810
Patrick Morgan
(617) 685–8061

Dallas, TX 75243
11969 Plano Rd., # 150
Craig Simmons, (214) 437–
  5151
AGJ

C. V. Mosby Co., Publisher
11830 Westline Industrial
  Dr.
St. Louis, MO 63146
Customer Service Dept.
(800) 325–4177
(314) 872–8370

Mountain Medical
    Equipment, Inc.
10488 West Centennial Rd.
Littleton, CO 80127
Judy Stechert
(800) 525–8950
(303) 973–1200

MPCS Video Industries,
    Inc.
514 W. 57th St.
New York, NY 10019
Max Meyerson
(212) 586–3690

Multi-Media Publishing,
    Inc.
1393 South Inca St.
Denver, CO 80223
Merv Leamon
(303) 778–1404

N

John Nageldinger & Son,
    Inc.
210 Post Avenue
Westbury, NY 11590
Dan Etzold
(800) 645–3496
(516) 997–6770

Narco Scientific
330 Jacksonville Rd.
Hatboro, PA 19040
Joe Moffett
(215) 675–5200

N.A.R.D.A., Inc.
F & M Bldg., Suite 600
West Chester, PA 19380
C. J. Rudderow
(215) 696–7691

NASCO
901 Janesville Ave.
Ft. Atkinson, WI 53538
Gary Allen
(414) 563–2446

National Catheter Co.
Hook Rd.
Argyle, NY 12801
Marketing/Sales Dept.
(518) 638–8232
(518) 638–8237

National Laboratories
225 Summit Ave.
Montvale, NJ 07642
Service Center
(201) 391–8500

National Medical
    Specialties
6900 Aragon Circle
Buena Park, CA 90620
Wayne Laird
(714) 522–5850
BH

Nellcor, Incorporated
25495 Whitesell St.
Hayward, CA 94545
(415) 887–5858

Nephron Corp.
3319 Pacific Ave.
Tacoma, WA 98401
John Bigler
(800) 426–3603
(206) 475–3452

KNF Neuberger, Inc.
P.O. Box 4060
Princeton, NJ 08540
Tony Innamorato
(609) 799–4350

Newport Medical
    Instruments, Inc.
300 N. Newport Blvd.
Newport Beach, CA 92663
Doug Domurat
(714) 642–3910

Norton Health Care
    Products
P.O. Box 350
Akron, OH 44309

North American Drager
148B Quarry Rd.
Telford, PA 18969
Thomas W. Barford
(215) 723–9824

North American Instrument
    Corp.
P.O. Box 350
48 Pine S.
Glens Falls, NY 12801
(518) 747–4171

Nova Biomedical
200 Prospect St.
Waltham, MA 02254
Barbara Callaham
(617) 894–0800

Nova Medical, Inc.
620 South B St., Suite A
Tustin, CA 92680
Marilyn Foreman
(714) 544–7711

Novametrix Medical
    Systems, Inc.
1 Barnes Industrial Park
    Rd. S.
Wallingford, CT 06492
Jay Zebora
(800) 243–3444

Nova-VentRx, Inc.
500 Glenn Ave.
Wheeling, IL 60090
Bernard R. Paluch
(312) 541–4222

Nursing Abstracts Co., Inc.
P.O. Box 295
Forest Hills, NY 11375
A. Buchsbaum

O

O & J Electronics, Inc.
See Datamed Corporation

OEM Medical, Inc.
8741 Landmark Rd.
Richmond, VA 23228
Bill Yates
(800) 572–2040
(804) 264–7691

Ohio Medical Products
See Ohmeda

Ohmeda
3030 Airco Dr.
P.O. Box 7550
Madison, WI 53707
(608) 221–1551

Olympic Medical
440 Seventh Ave. S.
Seattle, WA 98108
Dorothy Butcher
(800) 426–0353

Oxequip Health Industries
12601 S. Springfield Ave.
Chicago, IL 60658
Customer Service
(312) 371–3500

Oxford Medical, Inc.
11526 53rd St. N.
Clearwater, FL 33520
Jeff Olseth
(813) 577–4500

Oximetrix, Inc.
1212 Terra Bella Ave.
Mountain View, CA 94043
Customer Service
  Department
(415) 961–4380

Oxygen Enrichment
  Company, Ltd.
P.O. Box 1025
Schenectady, NY 12301
(518) 374–4111

Oxy Med, Inc.
9145 Deering Ave.
Chatsworth, CA 91311
Michael Patterson
(213) 882–3726

P

Pacer Industries
8201 Sovereign Row
Dallas, TX 75247
Margaret Parker
(800) 874–9090
(214) 637–4600

Pall Biomedical Products
  Corp.
2200 Northern Blvd.
East Hills, NY 11548
Sam Worthon
(800) 645–6578

Parke-Davis
Div. of Warner-Lambert
  Co.
201 Tabor Road
Morris Plains, NJ 07950
Jack Temco
(201) 540–2000

Parks Medical Electronics
P.O. Box 5669
Aloha, OR 97006
L. Parks
(800) 547–6427

Passy & Muir, Inc.
4521 Campus Dr., # 273
Irvine, CA 92715
Patricia Passy
(714) 974–5313

Patient Technology, Inc.
400 Rabro Dr.
Hauppauge, NY 11788
(516) 582–5900

Peace Medical, Inc.
17 Beaumont Terr.
West Orange, NJ 07052
(201) 731–5185

Penox Technologies, Inc.
1 Penox Plaza
Pittston, PA 18740
Michael Downend
(800) 233–3029
(717) 655–1421

Perkin-Elmer
2771 N. Garey Avenue
Pomona, CA 91767
Urie McCleary, Jr.
(714) 593–3581

Physio Parameters
P.O. Box 1297
Reseda, CA 91335
Lynnie Hart
(213) 342–8236

Plas-Met Corporation
516 Lunt Ave.
Schaumburg, IL 60193
Douglas M. Kendon
(312) 893–5777

Pneumatronics, Inc.
676 W. Wilson Ave.
Glendale, CA 91203
Donald R. Casas
(213) 247–4711

Polamedco, Inc.
1625 17th St.
Santa Monica, CA 90404
Albert L. Harrison
(213) 450–1396

Portex, Inc.
42 Industrial Way
Wilmington, MA 01887
(617) 658–5110

J. T. Posey Co.
5635 Peck Road
Arcadia, CA 91006
Stan or Claria
(800) 423–4292
(818) 443–3143

Precision Metering, Inc.
237–21 Fairbury Avenue
Bellerose, NY 11426
Stephen J. Dolan
(212) 343–9841

Prescription Air
G7503 Fenton Road
P.O. Box 438
Grand Blanc, MI 48439
Doug Thomas

Prescription Air of Indiana
5933 Stoney Creek Dr.
Fort Wayne, IN 46825
Bob Dawson
(219) 424–4423

Prins Medical Design
P.O. Box 341
Newbury Park, CA 91320
Jim Prins
(805) 499–3216

PRN
See Mediq/PRN

Professional Instruments
P.O. Box 767
Glendale, CA 91209
Cliff Carroll
(213) 845–5434

**Professional Medical
    Equipment Services, Inc.**
812 Rock Lane
Blue Springs, MO 64015
Tom Richardson
(816) 229–7707

**Professional Tape Company,
    Inc.**
144 Tower Dr.
Burr Ridge, IL 60521
Randy Zehr
(312) 986–1800

Proto-Med, Inc.
5360 Manhattan Circle
Boulder, CO 80303
John Sichel
(800) 821–9690
(303) 494–0050

**Pulmonary Care Services,
    Inc.**
11880 Bird Rd., Suite 319
Miami, FL 33175
J. Gregory Anderson
(305) 442–8117

**Puritan-Bennett
    Corporation**
9401 Indian Creek Pkwy.,
Bldg. 40
P.O. Box 25905
Overland Park, KS 66225–
5905

Pyramid Film & Video
P.O. Box 1048
Santa Monica, CA 90406
Teresa Morrissey
(213) 828–7577

Q

Quinton Instrument Co.
2121 Terry Avenue
Seattle, WA 98121
Customer Service
(800) 426–0538
(206) 223–7373

**QuinTron Instrument Co.,
    Inc.**
3712 W. Pierce St.
Milwaukee, WI 53215
Lou Betzwieser
(414) 645–1515

R

Radiometer America, Inc.
811 Sharon Drive
Westlake, OH 44145
Donald O. Reiss
(216) 871–8900

Ramcom, Inc.
Distribution Center
713 Chapel Road
North Hills, PA 19038
Administrative Offices
1110 Norwalk Road
Philadelphia, PA 19115
Donna K. Ryderr
(215) 572–7711

Rely-On Medical Industries
5120 NE 12th Avenue
Ft. Lauderdale, FL 33334
David E. Smith
(305) 772–8442

**Research Development
    Corp.**
2225 Palou
San Francisco, CA 94124
Duane Hardy

Research Plus, Inc.
P.O. Box 324
Bayonne, NJ 07002
(201) 823–3592

Respiratory Care, Inc.
900 West University Drive
Arlington Heights, IL
    60004
Renee Wolanski
(312) 259–7400

**Respiratory Care Services,
    Inc.**
P.O. Drawer 9366
5135 Galaxie Drive
Jackson, MS 39206
Director of Human
    Resources
(601) 982–8843

**Respiratory Management
    Services, Inc. (RMS)**
364 Adams St.
Bedford Hills, NY 10507
Suzanne McCue
(800) 431–2460
(914) 666–2990
(212) 379–7744

Respiratory West
15 Varsity Court
Ventura, CA 93003
Vern Arnold
(805) 644–3607

Respironics, Inc.
650 Seco Road
Monroeville, PA 15146
(800) 245–2767
(412) 373–8114

Respitrace Corp.
731 Saw Mill River Road
Ardsley, NY 10502
Anita Boehme
(914) 693–9240

Respitron, Inc.
430 Mill Hill Avenue
Bridgeport, CT 06610
Stan Siwicki

Res-Support, Inc.
P.O. Box 2082
Corvallis, OR 97330
Jean F. Rosendahl
(503) 758–1151

R. E. Reynolds Co., Inc.
121 Park Avenue
Rochester, NY 14607
Norma Reynolds
(716) 271–8890

Riker Laboratories, Inc.
19901 Nordhoff St.
Northridge, CA 91326
(213) 341–1300

R & L Products, Inc.
P.O. Box 1867
Richardson, TX 75080
Ronald G. Wilke
(214) 690–9147

RMP Co
6831 Uppingham Road
Fayetteville, NC 28306
(919) 424–1133

Robertshaw Controls Co.
333 N. Euclid Way
Anaheim, CA 92803
Richard C. Rodriguez
(714) 535–8151

**Roche Medical Electronics,
    Inc.**
Brickyard Road
Cranbury, NJ 08512
(800) 257–5110

Rodder Instrument
775 Sunshine Drive
Los Altos, CA 94022
J. Rodder
(415) 968–4708

Rolof Enterprises
3772 Lockland Dr., Suite
    20
Los Angeles, CA 90008
Anthony Williams

Ross Laboratories
625 Cleveland Ave.
Columbus, OH 43216
Trish Caldwalder
(614) 227–3333

Roxane Laboratories, Inc.
330 Oak Street
Columbus, OH 43216
(614) 228–5403

R2 Corp.
5422 West Touhy Avenue
Skokie, IL 60077
(312) 673–8400

Hans Rudolph Inc.
7200 Wyandotte St.
Kansas City, MO 64114
John Rudolph
(816) 363–5522

**Rush-Hampton Industries,
    Inc.**
P.O. Box 3000
3000 Industrial Drive
Longwood, FL 32750
Brenda Joiner
(305) 831–5200

S

Safety Medical Corp.
800 Chester Pike
Sharon Hill, PA 19079
John R. Kennedy
(215) 534–3500

Safeway Products, Inc.
440 Middlefield St.
Middletown, CT 06457
H. B. Hall
(203) 346–6601

Salter Labs
P.O. Box 608
Arvin, CA 93203
Peter W. Salter
(800) 235–4203
In CA (800) 421–0024

W. B. Saunders Co.
W. Washington Sq.
Philadelphia, PA 19010
(215) 574–4700

Schuco
Div. of American Caduceus
    Industries, Inc.
201 Hillside Avenue
P.O. Box 246
Williston Park, NY 11596
Customer Service
(800) 645–2500
(516) 741–7100

Scitec Corp.
5680 S. Syracuse Circle
Suite 300
Englewood, CO 80110
Jeffrey Butler
(303) 741–3488

Seal-Seat Company
1200 Monterey Pass Rd.
Monterey Park, CA 91754–
    3617
Tom Lynch
(213) 269–1311

**Seamless Hospital Products
    Company, Inc.**
Barnes Industrial Park No.
    Box 828
Wallingford, CT 06492
Gary V. Halick
(800) 243–3030
(203) 265–7671

Sechrist Industries, Inc.
2820 Gretta Lane
Anaheim, CA 92806
Bob Pearson
(714) 630–2400

SensorMedics Corp.
1630 S. State College Blvd.
Anaheim, CA 92806
Steve Cornet
(800) 231–2466
(800) 821–8145
In Canada (800) 325–6024
In Europe (022) 553344
(714) 634–0233

Sensors, Inc.
Subsidiary of Dynatech
    Corp.
6812 So. State Rd.
Saline, MI 48176
(800) 247–7038
In MI (800) 722–4153

Sheridan Catheter Corp.
Route 40
Argyle, NY 12809
R. S. Wallace
(518) 638–6101

Sherwood Medical
Argyle Division
1831 Olive St.
St. Louis, MO 63103
Jim Brooks
(314) 241–5700

Anaheim, CA, 1620 S.
Lewis St., (714) 634–
2711, Branch
Dallas, TX, 3551 Dan
Morton Dr., (214) 296–
2512, Branch
Decatur, GA, 2525 Park
Central, (404) 981–
8721, Branch
Elgin, IL, 875 Toll Gate
Rd. (312) 695–4070,
Branch
N. Brunswick, NJ, 1605
Jersey Ave., (201) 846–
6630,
Branch

Shiley Inc.
17600 Gillette Ave.
Irvine, CA 92714
Linda Thompson
(714) 250–0500

**Siemens-Elema Ventilator
Systems**
2360 No. Palmer Dr.
Schaumberg, IL 60195
Christer Hellsten
(312) 397–5975

**S.L.O. Health Products,
Inc.**
1155 Fifth St.
Los Osos, CA 93402
John S. Mauro, Jr.
(805) 528–3197

S & M Instrument Co.
202 Airport Blvd.
Doylestown, PA 18901
Bill Letvenko or
Mark Eisentock
(215) 345–9232

**SoloPak Laboratories/
MPL, Inc.**
1820 West Roscoe St.
Chicago, IL 60657
S. De Prizio
(312) 248–3810

Sontek Medical, Inc.
P.O. Box 459
31 Fletcher Avenue
Lexington, MA 02173
Terry L. Crabtree
(617) 863–1410

S.O.S. Oxygen Service, Inc.
25 South "H" Street
Lake Worth, FL 33460
David E. Smith
(305) 588–8574

Source Medical, Inc.
P.O. Box 6106
Bridgewater, NJ 08807
(201) 231–0123

**Southeastern Pennsylvania
Respiratory Inc.**
P.O. Box 322
Exton, PA 19341
Frank Dunigan
(215) 363–8300

Spacelabs, Inc.
4200 150th NE
P.O. Box 97013
Redmond, WA 98073–9713
(206) 882–3700

Spirometrics, Inc.
26 Essex St.
Andover, MA 01810
Paula Kelly
(800) 235–0004
(617) 470–1872

Spirotech, Inc.
3772 Pleasantdale Road
Suite 100
Atlanta, GA 30340
J. Richard Glymph
(404) 938–6300

Spital Medical, Inc.
P.O. Box 91
Inkster, MI 48141
Barry E. Horne
(313) 278–8544

The Sporicidin Co.
4000 Massachusetts Ave.
NW
Washington, DC 20016
Warren L. Cook, Jr.
(202) 244–6606

Sterilaire Medical, Inc.
620 South "B" St.
Tustin, CA 92680
Bob Foreman
(714) 544–7711

Strom Corporation
121 Lewisville Center,
158
Lewisville, TX 75067
Betty C. Strom
(214) 221–3564

Stuart Pharmaceutical
Div. of ICI Americas, Inc.
Wilmington, DE 19897
John Hazlett

Sumetrix, Inc.
Medical Systems Div.
25455 Barton Rd., Suite
207B
P.O. Box 963
Loma Linda, CA 92354
(714) 796–0111

Sunnydale Industries, Inc.
RR #2
Centralia, MO 65240
Lester Halvorsen
(314) 682–2128

Superior Plastic Products Corp.
Cumberland Industrial Park
Cumberland, RI 02864
Marshall, Kim, or Liz
(800) 556–6462

Surgikos, Inc.
P.O. Box 130
Arlington, TX 76010
Customer Service
(800) 433–5009
(817) 273–5895

Survival Technology, Inc.
8101 Glenbrook Rd.
Bethesda, MD 20814
Nancy H. Mancuso
(800) 638–8093
(301) 656–5600

Sybron Corp.
Medical Products Div.
P.O. Box 23077
Rochester, NY 14692
John E. Mooney
(716) 271–6060

T

Technical Trading Center, Inc.
122 E. Main St.
Little Falls, NJ 07424
John Shakarijan
(201) 256–1035

TeleDiagnostic Systems
515 Spruce St.
San Francisco, CA 94118
Donald Bale
(800) 227–3224
(415) 221–3000

Telemed Cardio-Pulmonary Systems
See Tenet Information Services

Telesensory Systems, Inc.
P.O. Box 10099
Palo Alto, CA 94304
(415) 493–2626

Tenet Information Services
5181 South Third West
Salt Lake City, UT 84107
William Nicholls
(801) 268–3840

Tensor
P.O. Box 153449
Irving, TX 75015
Robert Succi
(214) 986–1580

Terumo Corporation
2805 E. Ana St.
Compton, CA 90221
John Schwartz
(213) 537–3510
120 New England Ave.
Piscataway, NJ 08854
Ronald M. Loomis
(800) 526–3531
(201) 463–1315

Thieme-Stratton, Inc.
381 Park Ave. South
New York, NY 10016
J. Kemp Passano
(212) 683–5091

Thompson Respiration Products
See Puritan-Bennett Corp.,
Portable Ventilator Div.

Timeter Instrument Corp.
See the Timeter Group

The Timeter Group
2501 Oregon Pike
Lancaster, PA 17601
Rosanne M. Donahue
(717) 569–2695

Timeter International, Inc.
2501 Oregon Pike
Lancaster, PA 17601
Greg Nielson
(717) 569–2695
Telex 466816 TIM LNS C1

Total Medical Systems
7161 Engineer Road
San Diego, CA 92111
Larry Westfall
(714) 560–5771

Transtracheal Systems
601 E. 18th Ave., # 200
Denver, CO 80203
Rae Reynolds
(800) 527–2667
(303) 839–1119

Travenol Laboratories, Inc.
Medical Products Division
1 Baxter Parkway
Deerfield, IL 60015
Dennis Emmer
(312) 940–5550

Traverse Medical Monitors
6812 S. State Rd.
Saline, MI 48176
William T. Baker
(800) 247–7038
In MI (800) 722–4153
(313) 429–2100

Tri-Anim Health Services, Inc.
1630 Flower St.
Glendale, CA 91201
Dan Pister
(800) TRI-ANIM
(818) 247–9187

Tri Med Inc.
13240 Northup Way
Bellevue, WA 98005
Jon Stuart
(800) 558–2345

Tri W-G, Inc.
215–12th Ave., N.E.
Valley City, ND 58072
Frank H. Erling
(800) 437–8011

T. T. C., Inc.
122 E. Main St.
Little Falls, NJ 07424
International Division
(201) 256–1035
Telex: 710–988–5714

U

U-Line Products
P.O. Box 65736
Los Angeles, CA 90065
J. Ulman
(213) 223–7663

Union Carbide Corp.
4801 West 16th Street
Indianapolis, IN 46224
Paul O'Rourke
(800) 238–5055

United Ad Label Co., Inc.
P.O. Box 2165
Whittier, CA 90610
Suzi Molina
(800) 423–4643
In CA (800) 352–4345

UO Equipment Co.
5859 W. 34th St.
Houston, TX 77092
Bob Wright, Jr.
(713) 686–1869

Utah Medical Products
7043 South 300 W.
P.O. Box 9
Midvale, UT 84047
Darla Gill
(800) 533–4984
(601) 566–1200

V

Vacumed
2261 Palma Dr.
Ventura, CA 93003–5789
Ron Thompson or Craig
Vivas
(800) 235–3333
(805) 644–7461

Vaisala Inc.
22 Cummings Park
Woburn, MA 01801
Marketing Dept.
(617) 933–4500

Validyne Engineering Corp.
8626 Wilbur Avenue
Northridge, CA 91324
Application Engineering
(818) 886–2057

Vascular Technology, Inc.
108 Middlesex St.
N. Chelmsford, MA 01863
Bill Oliver
(617) 251–8977

Ventilation Associates
6800 Main, Suite 106B
Houston, TX 77030
Bob Peterson
(713) 526–3856

Ventco Medical Co., Inc.
1425 Dorchester, Canada
(514) 875–5744
Telex 055–60562
Senfin, MH
97 Lake Street
Rouses Point, New York
12979

Ventronics
Div. of Hudson Oxygen
27711 Diaz St.
P.O. Box 66
Temecula, CA 92390–0066
(800) 221–0338
In CA (800) 221–0338

Veriflo
2500 Canal Blvd.
Richmond, CA 94804
Dave Sapiane
(415) 235–9590

Vesta, Inc.
4380 S. Tenth St.
Milwaukee, WI 53221
Bob Olson
(414) 483–9090

Vickers Medical Products Corp.
U.S. Hwy. 22
P.O. Box 101
Whitehouse Station, NJ 08889
Nancy Wharmby
(800) 526–3949

Victor Equipment Co.
Medical Products Div.
Airport Rd.
P.O. Box 1007
Denton, TX 76202
Hal Olcott
(817) 566–2000

Video Digest of Continuing Medical Information
4 Militia Dr.
Lexington, MA 02173
Janice Emanuelson
(617) 861–0404

Vitalograph Medical Instrumentation
8347 Quivira Road
Lenexa, KS 66215
(800) 255–6626

Vital Signs Inc.
20 Campus Rd.
Totowa, NJ 07512
Paul Bennett
(800) 932–0760

Vitatron Systems, Inc.
201 E. Pine St.
Orlando, FL 32801
Rick Chambers
(305) 423–2221

W

Walton Laboratories
1 Carol Place
Moonachie, NJ 07074
Jay S. Speigel
(201) 641–5700

Wave Energy Systems, Inc.
30 W. 54th St., Suite 807
New York, NY 10019
(212) 765–1510

R. S. Weber & Associates
31240 La Baya Drive
Westlake Village, CA 91362
Jerry Birnbaum
(213) 889–4630

Welch Allyn, Inc.
4341 State Street Rd.
Skaneateles Falls, NY 13153
Kenneth P. Heinz
(315) 685–8351, ext. 515

Wescor, Inc.
459 South Main St.
Logan, UT 84321
Kent S. Thomas
(800) 453–2725

Western Enterprises
33672 Pin Oak Parkway
Avon Lake, OH 44012
Charles A. Rudd
(216) 933–2171

John Wiley & Sons, Inc., Publishers
605 Third Ave.
New York, NY 10158
Ida Kilroe
(212) 850–6000

Winthrop-Breon Laboratories Inc.
90 Park Avenue
New York, NY 10016
(212) 907–2000

Wyeth Laboratories
P.O. Box 8299
Philadelphia, PA 19101
T. E. Gallagher
(215) 688–4400

Y

Year Book Medical Publishers
35 East Wacker Drive
Chicago, IL 60601
(312) 726–9733

Yellow Springs Instrument Co., Inc.
P.O. Box 279
Yellow Springs, OH 45387
Richard Horn
(513) 767–7241

Appendix B

Position Statements of the American Association for Respiratory Care

Definition of Respiratory Care

Respiratory care is an allied health specialty employed with medical direction in the treatment, management, control, diagnostic evaluation and care of patients with deficiencies and abnormalities with the cardiopulmonary system.

Respiratory care shall mean the therapeutic use of the following: medical gases and administration apparatus, environmental control systems, humidification, aerosols, medications, ventilatory support, bronchopulmonary drainage, pulmonary rehabilitation, cardiopulmonary resuscitation and airway management.

Specific testing techniques are employed in respiratory care to assist in diagnosis, monitoring, treatment, and research. This shall be understood to include measurement of ventilatory volumes, pressures, flows, blood gas analysis and other related physiologic monitoring

Respiratory Care Scope of Practice

The practice of respiratory care encompasses activities in: diagnostic evaluation, therapy, and education of the patient, family and public. These activities are supported by education, research and administration.

Diagnostic activities include but are not limited to: (1) obtaining and analyzing physiological specimens; (2) interpreting physiological data; (3) performing tests and studies of the cardiopulmonary system; (4) performing neurophysiological studies, and (5) performing sleep disorder studies.

Therapy includes but is not limited to application and monitoring of: (1) medical gases (excluding anesthetic gases) and environmental control systems; (2) mechanical ventilatory support, (3) artificial airway care; (4) bronchopulmonary hygiene; (5) pharmacological agents related to respiratory care procedures; (6) cardiopulmonary rehabilitation; and (7) hemodynamic cardiovascular support.

The focus of patient and family education activities is to promote knowledge of disease process, medical therapy and self help. Public education activities focus on the promotion of cardiopulmonary wellness.

Statement of Principles

The American Association for Respiratory Care (AARC), a national society of heath care professionals, is sponsored by the American College of Chest Physicians, the American Society of Anesthesiologists, and the American Thoracic Society.* The Association is dedicated to maintaining the highest standards of practice in respiratory care.

Respiratory care is defined as a health care specialty under medical direction in the assessment, treatment, management, control, diagnostic evaluation, and care of patients with deficiencies and abnormalities of the cardiopulmonary system.

Respiratory care shall mean the diagnostic and therapeutic use of the following: medical gases and administration apparatus, environmental control systems, humidification, aerosols, medications, ventilatory support, bronchopulmonary drainage, pulmonary rehabilitation, cardiopulmonary resuscitation and airway management.

Specific testing techniques are employed in respiratory care to assist in diagnosis, monitoring, treatment, and research of cardiopulmonary pathology. This shall be understood to include measurement of ventilatory volumes, airway pressures, gas flows, blood gas analysis, and other related physiologic monitoring.

The respiratory therapy technician and respiratory therapist are integral members of the hospital based health care team working under the supervision and guidance of a physician. They shall work together to determine appropriate diagnoses and administer appropriate treatment for acute and chronic pulmonary and cardiovascular disorders.

The AARC recognizes the need to assure high quality patient care at affordable cost. To that end, we believe a combination of specialized formal education and clinical training is the best method to develop highly skilled respiratory care personnel. The AARC endorses the standards of practice adopted by the Joint Commission on Accreditation of Hospitals as an additional quality assurance mechanism and sees uniform credentialing as another positive step toward assuring high quality health care.

The concept of peer review as a quality assurance mechanism is attractive to the AARC, and we strongly endorse efforts to develop various peer review programs which involve respiratory therapists and respiratory therapy technicians in audits and other review techniques.

Role Model Statement

As health care professionals engaged in the performance of cardiopulmonary care, the practitioners of this profession must strive to maintain the highest personal and professional standards. A most important standard in the profession is for that practitioner to serve as a role model in matters concerning health.

In addition to upholding the code of ethics of this profession by continually striving to render the highest quality of patient care possible, the respiratory care practitioner shall set himself apart as a leader and advocate of public respiratory health.

The respiratory care practitioner shall participate in activities leading to awareness of the causes and prevention of pulmonary disease and the problems associated with the cardiopulmonary system.

*Other sponsoring organizations include: American Academy of Pediatrics, American College of Allergists, and Society of Critical Care Medicine.

The respiratory care practitioner shall support the development and promotion of pulmonary disease awareness programs, to include smoking cessation programs, pulmonary function screenings, air pollution monitoring, allergy warning, and other public education programs.

The respiratory care practitioner shall support research in all areas where efforts could promote improved health and could prevent disease.

The respiratory care practitioner shall provide leadership in determining health promotion and disease prevention activities for students, faculty, practitioners, patients, and the general public.

The respiratory care practitioner shall serve as a physical example of cardiopulmonary health by abstaining from tobacco use and shall make a special personal effort to eliminate smoking and the use of other tobacco products from his home and work environment.

The respiratory care practitioner shall uphold himself as a model for all members of the health care team by demonstrating his responsibilities and shall cooperate with other health care professionals to meet the health needs of the public.

Official Definitions

Respiratory Care Specialist:

The following definitions are based on a classification of respiratory care specialist by education, experience, and professional credentialing.

Respiratory Therapist:

1. Graduate Respiratory Therapist: One who is a graduate of a respiratory therapist program approved by the Council on Medical Education of the American Medical Association.
2. Registered Respiratory Therapist: One who has been registered by the National Board for Respiratory Care (NBRC) (formerly American Registry of Inhalation Therapists).

Respiratory Therapy Technician:

1. Graduate Respiratory Therapy Technician:
   a. Effective until December 31, 1974: One who is a graduate of a respiratory therapy technician program designed to prepare candidates for certification, or, one who has received on-the-job training in respiratory care.
   b. Effective January 1, 1975: One who is a graduate of a respiratory therapy technician program approved by the Council on Medical Education of the American Medical Association.
2. Certified Respiratory Therapy Technician: One who has been certified by the National Board for Respiratory Care (NBRC) (formerly administered by the Technician Certification Board (TCB), (AARC).

Respiratory Therapy Assistant:

1. Respiratory Therapy Assistant: (Effective January 1, 1975: One who has received on-the-job training in respiratory care.

Student:

1. Respiratory Therapy Student: One who is enrolled in a program which follows the essentials for an approved respiratory care program as established by the American Medical Association's Council on Medical Education.

2. Respiratory Therapy Trainee: One who is employed by a Joint Commission on Accreditation of Hospitals (JCAH) approved medical facility in the respiratory service while receiving on-the-job training as a respiratory therapy assistant.

Respiratory Home Care

Respiratory home care is defined as those forms of respiratory care provided in the patient's place of residence by personnel trained in respiratory care working under medical supervision. The respiratory therapist and respiratory therapy technician, who are part of a comprehensive interdisciplinary team of health professionals by virtue of their specialized training and expertise, are key members for the success of a respiratory home care program.

The goals of respiratory home care are to improve the patient's physical well-being, potential for productivity, and to promote self-sufficiency within the individual's limitations. The role of the respiratory therapist and respiratory therapy technician is to provide their expertise in the areas of administration of therapy, equipment use and care, patient and family education and instruction, and patient monitoring and evaluation.

Standards for Respiratory Home Care

Definition

Respiratory home care is defined as those forms of respiratory care provided in the patient's place of residence by personnel trained in respiratory care working under medical supervision.

Patients with airway obstruction and other respiratory afflictions, because of the chronic nature of their disease, require comprehensive and continuous care. Examples include: chronic obstructive pulmonary disease (COPD) or chronic air flow obstruction, asthma, chronic bronchitis, emphysema, cystic fibrosis, chronic interstitial lung disease or fibrosis, asbestosis, anthracosilicosis, byssinosis, berylliosis or other pneumoconioses, poliomyelitis or other restrictive disorders, and any other chronic condition affecting gas transport or causing dyspnea, cough, sputum production, or other disability. In many cases, especially when ambulation is restricted or equipment is used, home care is indicated.

Some aspects of respiratory home care for COPD patients are under study and are debatable, but much evidence throughout the years supports the role of home care in assisting the individual to stay alive, to maintain or improve functional ability in activities of daily living and employment, and to reduce acute hospitalization.

The goals of qualified respiratory home care are to support life in some instances, in others to improve the patient's physical, emotional, and social well-being and productivity, to promote patient and family self-sufficiency within their limitations, to provide respiratory care of high quality under medical supervision, and to ensure cost effectiveness of respiratory therapy modalities.

Standard I

The need for therapy must be clearly established. There must be criteria and therapeutic objectives for program entry requirements. A unified approach should exist between the physician and therapist for the objectives and modalities of therapy.

Discussion

Before respiratory home care is provided, there must be a reasonable expectation that the therapy will be of benefit. The physician is expected to provide information that will serve to establish that the patient actually has a cardiopulmonary condition that can be properly treated in the home setting. The physician shall agree to therapeutic objectives established for the home care patient, to the modalities to be used in reaching these objectives, and shall direct the therapy regime. Home care team members shall evaluate the conditions, abilities, and progress of the patient and report these in the medical record for suitable evaluation. If the patient is in the hospital and it is determined that home care is to be provided then there must be adequate discharge planning by a designated individual or group.

This should expedite the procurement of any home care appliances, and when possible, pre-discharge evaluation to determine whether the patient can use and benefit from the therapy.

Home care services are provided ideally by a team of health care professionals whose membership and roles depend on the needs of the patient. By virtue of their specialized training and expertise, the respiratory therapist and respiratory therapy technician are key members of this team. Other members may be physicians, nurses, physical therapists, social workers, etc. There is often no clear boundary between respiratory care services, nursing, physical therapy, and other professional roles.

Standard II

A medical record that includes the prescription must be established and maintained on all patients receiving any form of respiratory home care.

Discussion

Respiratory care may not be given without written prescription of the patient's own physician. The type of equipment, frequency, duration of therapy, medication (including dosage and dilution ratio), and any precautions, must be included. All services rendered shall be documented in the medical record, including the type of therapy, date and time of administration, effects of therapy, any adverse reactions, and documentation of patient education.

The responsible physician shall document in the patient's medical record the pertinent diagnosis and a timely, pertinent clinical evaluation of the overall results of respiratory care, based on objective and subjective evidence and shall document any modifications of therapy as a result of the evaluation.

The provider department, company (supplier), or home health agency shall maintain a record of the prescription, patient's progress, visits, equipment maintenance, and cost, available upon each home visit and upon transfer. A copy will be forwarded at least quarterly to the doctor.

Standard III

Respiratory care equipment used must be safe and appropriate. The patient must demonstrate its effective use, and he or his family its proper maintenance, including sterilization or appropriate cleanliness.

Discussion

In not every case is equipment necessary as part of respiratory home care. In many cases, bronchopulmonary drainage procedures performed by respiratory therapists, physical therapists, nurses, or family members may suffice to meet objectives. Equipment, when provided, shall meet all safety standards, and be appropriate for its intended use.*

The patient, family, or significant other person must demonstrate ability to maintain, operate, clean, and disinfect any respiratory care equipment used. The patient or person administering any medication must demonstrate its safe use and a knowledge of side effects and what to do if they develop. If necessary, there must be a full explanation of other precautionary measures. Repair and technical service or backup equipment should be available on a 24-hour emergency basis. Both rental and purchase of respiratory equipment used at home should be available. Financial options regarding equipment rental or purchase should be revealed to the patient.

Documentation of patient education, equipment use and maintenance, and evaluation of cost effectiveness shall be provided in the medical record. The current medical literature suggests that there is questionable efficacy of IPPB or other mechanical aids on stable COPD. Therefore, it is incumbent on the prescribing physician to justify rationale and expenditure of such equipment. The appropriate use of home oxygen should also be documented by objective means.

Standard IV

There must be evidence that patients are receiving follow-up evaluations at least once per month, and more often if necessary, by some member of the home care team.

Discussion

During the initial instruction session, future needs and visits should be based on need rather than preestablished number of visits which may be unnecessary. However, all patients on home therapy should be visited at least monthly. When possible, it is desirable that the physician perform at least some of the visits. A visiting nurse, when used, should be a full member of the respiratory home care team. The respiratory home care program must be under observation and evaluation at all times to determine and maintain the therapeutic value of the home care program. A recommendation should be made to the physician to discontinue the program when the patient's needs are not met.

Ethical Performance of Respiratory Home Care

The Standards for Respiratory Home Care established by the American Association for Respiratory Care (AARC) and published in the November, 1979 issue of Respiratory Care (24:1080–82, 1979) are still relevant and remain in force.

Confusion still exists, however, concerning home care practices. Specifically, ambiguous examples of potential conflicts of interest and alleged violations of employee/employer relations have been published. Although these examples were published in an attempt to clarify the issue of ethical home care practice, such has not been the result.

In response to numerous inquiries from practitioners as to what constitutes ethical arrangements for provision of home care, the Standards Committee is defining concisely what shall be

*See NFPA Pamphlet # 56Hm "Manual for the Home Use of Respiratory Therapy," National Fire Protection Association, Batterymarch Park, Boston, MA 02269.

considered as a conflict of interest. First, the Code of Ethics of the AARC applies to all respiratory care practices regardless of the environment in which care may be delivered. In general, the following definition of conflict of interest is provided.

Under no circumstances should any respiratory care practitioner engage in any activity which compromises the motive for the provision of any therapy procedures, the advice or counsel given patients and/or families, or in any manner profit from referral arrangements with home care providers.

Specifically, for the purposes of this document, conflict of interest shall be defined as: Any act of a respiratory care practitioner during or outside the practitioner's principal employment for which the practitioner receives any form of consideration for:

a) The referral of patients to specific home care providers.
b) The solicitation of others for specific home care provider referrals.
c) Recommendations for ordering of specific therapy procedures and/or equipment.
d) Recommendations for the continuation of unwarranted procedures and/or equipment.
e) The association of any practitioner with any home care provder, when profit or revenue generation influences the selection, evaluation, or continuation of any home care procedure and/or equipment.
f) Individuals who are either employed by or receive remuneration from both health care institutions which may refer patients and by durable medical equipment suppliers who offer respiratory home care must openly disclose this relationship to both parties.
g) Institutionally based respiratory care practitioners who have significant ownership interest in a durable medical equipment company which provides respiratory home care must openly disclose this relationship to the employing institution, Medicare Part B carriers, and all others who may be involved in the referral process. The therapist must remove himself from the process of patient referrals to that provider.

Awareness of activities that may be viewed as being a conflict of interest and in violation of the Code of Ethics of the AARC shall be documented and sent to the Judicial Committee of the AARC, AARC Executive Office, 1720 Regal Row, #112, Dallas, Texas 75235.*

Statement of Principles on Fraud and Abuse in Home Care

Respiratory care is an important element in home health care for many patients. The relationship between durable medical equipment providers and respiratory care practitioners in the home care setting has occasionally led to improprieties by both parties. This is due principally to the ability of the institutional based respiratory care practitioners to influence durable medical equipment provider business and the financial solicitation of this influence by some durable medical equipment providers. The absence of direct reimbursement by third party payors for home care services provided by respiratory care practitioners contributes to this dilemma. The resulting improprieties range from elusive conflicts of interest to outright fraud and abuse as defined in the Medicare/Medicaid Anti-Fraud and Abuse Amendments of 1977 PL 95–142.

---

*Respiratory care practitioners must realize that any liability coverage provided by a primary employer does not necessarily extend to activities that are not directly related to that primary work.

The American Association for Respiratory Care is opposed to all forms of fraud and abuse and conflict of interest in respiratory home care. It is our position that:

1. Profit or revenue generation must not influence the selection, evaluation, or continuation of any respiratory home care services. Fees, kickbacks, or other remunerations paid or offered by durable medical equipment providers or received or solicited by respiratory care practitioners for referral of patients are considered unethical and illegal.
2. Individuals who are either employed by or receive remuneration from both health care institutions which may refer patients and by durable medical equipment suppliers who offer respiratory home care must openly disclose this relationship to both parties.
3. Institutionally based respiratory care practitioners who have significant ownership interest in a durable medical equipment company which provides respiratory home care must openly disclose this relationship to the employing institution, Medicare Part B carriers, and all others who may be involved in the referral process. The therapist must remove himself from the process of patient referrals to that provider.

The American Association for Respiratory Care fully supports this position and pledges to encourage its members to comply with this statement. Furthermore, we will cooperate with Federal and state law enforcement authorities to assist in assuring full compliance by durable medical equipment suppliers and respiratory care practitioners.

Index